Seeds of Light

HEALING MEDITATIONS FOR BODY AND SOUL

Elizabeth K. Stratton, M.S.

A FIRESIDE BOOK
Published by Simon & Schuster

FIRESIDE
Rockefeller Center
1230 Avenue of the Americas
New York, NY 10020

Copyright © 1997 by Elizabeth K. Stratton, M.S.

First Fireside Edition 1998

FIRESIDE and colophon are registered trademarks of Simon & Schuster Inc.

Designed by Irving Perkins Associates, Inc.

Manufactured in the United States of America

1 3 5 7 9 10 8 6 4 2

The Library of Congress has cataloged the Simon & Schuster edition as follows:
Stratton, Elizabeth K.
Seeds of light : healing meditations for body and soul /
Elizabeth K. Stratton.
p.   cm.
1. Healing—Religious aspects—Meditations.   I. Title.
BL65.M4S77   1997
291.4'32—dc21   96–54827
CIP
ISBN 0-684-83094-9
ISBN 0-684-83876-1 (Pbk)

For Charles Francis Bowden
he planted seeds of light in the hearts of many stars
now his star shines brightly in the Heart of God

Contents

INTRODUCTION

Planting Seeds
of Healing Energy

*A*ll life on Earth has grown from a tiny seed of potential. Each of us began as a fertilized egg, with the power of Creation directing our development. If physicists are correct, and the universe is composed primarily of light energy, then we are all seeds of light in the eyes of God, our Creator. God's seed of creative light within us is what transforms that egg into a fetus, newborn, child, and adult. Our bodies vibrate with this light energy, our hearts beat with its love, our souls interact with its Divinity, and our minds have the power to co-operate in creating new life from its power.

This book of healing meditations will help you plant seeds of light in your body, heart, soul, and daily life. They also will help you facilitate healing in other people.

As a spiritual healer, I see my main goal as helping each person to awaken the healer within: the combination of physical, emotional, mental, and spiritual energies that God has given to us. When used together, these energies create a powerful healing force that can strengthen the immune system, heal emotional wounds, generate forgiveness, protect us from negative energies, develop new perspectives on life, and deepen our relationship with our Creator. For the past twenty years, I have been designing healing meditations for my patients, students, family, friends, and even myself. Each person who has come to me, and each class I have taught, has given me an opportunity to use a healing meditation or to create a new one specifically designed for that situation.

Styles of Meditation

Most forms of meditation are based in the imagination. Imagination is a very useful tool. When people make statements like "That's only imaginary" or "It's all in your imagination," they think they are being derogatory and saying that something is illusory. But the imagination is the creative medium through which we live most of our lives. We are constantly imaging everything we think about and all the actions that we take. When students in my workshops or TOUCHING SPIRIT® Training Program tell me that they have trouble imaging, or can't image, I ask them what they had for breakfast. They can always tell me. What did *you* have for breakfast? How do you know? Because you can see it, right? The memory is accessed through imagery. If you want to reach over and pick up a glass of water, what happens to allow you to do that? You first have the thirst, then the desire to act, and the image of a glass of water. That image is what gets transferred from your brain through your central nervous system and into the nerves in your arm and hand. This transfer of image into energy into action is what allows you to pick up the glass of water.

This process of imaging *is* imagination, and can be used in an intentional way to create healing. If the imagination is directed through the use of specific images, then we called it *guided imagery*. If we begin with an initial direction or intention in a meditation, and then allow our unconscious to free flow with whatever images and information it wishes to produce, then we call it *creative visualization*.

From the Hindu and Buddhist traditions of meditation designed to open energy centers *(chakras)* and produce altered states of consciousness, to the Judeo-Christian use of prayer and contemplation to deepen one's relationship with God, and Dr. Carl Simonton's use of guided imagery in the 1970s to help cancer patients, there have been many styles and techniques of inner healing.

The most well-known is *relaxation:* By closing the eyes, breathing deeply, and progressively relaxing all the muscles, you sometimes can lower blood pressure, release headaches and migraines, reduce physical pain, and produce a general sense of well-being. "Deep Relaxation" is also a good meditation to use before doing any of the other meditations. It stills the rational mind and creates a state of deep calm that allows all meditations to work more effectively.

Some meditations are what I call *opening* meditations: They open certain energies within the subtle and physical bodies. The *subtle energy body* is the invisible energy field within and around the physical body. It is also called the *etheric body*, and it is the electromagnetic field of life force that keeps us alive. "Opening the Chakras with Color" directs your awareness to the seven centers of energy within the subtle energy body. When these centers are restricted in some way, the energies cannot flow in a balanced and healthy pattern. This condition can eventually lead to physical and emotional dis-ease. The meditation directs our awareness to these centers and assists us in opening the flow of subtle energies within and between the chakras.

Another kind of meditation is *insight* meditation: any kind of meditative process that provides new and healing insight into a specific condition or issue. For example, "Communicating with Your Body" allows you to change roles, as well as dialogue, with a physical symptom or illness in order to understand it better. This communication can provide new insight into the origin of the condition, and what is needed for healing to take place.

Affirmations are positive statements that, combined with *guided imagery* in a meditation, can help change negative beliefs into life-affirming ones. In "Psychic Self-Defense Affirmations," you begin by visualizing an old or recurrent situation that makes you feel vulnerable, and then shift this feeling of vulnerability into one of protection by adding new positive beliefs and images.

Mindfulness meditation can be practiced by paying close attention to whatever you are feeling or doing in the moment. You allow yourself to become as conscious as possible of how you are experiencing physical, emotional, mental, and spiritual reality. You watch your mind and where it goes, what it thinks; you notice the emotions you are feeling; and you pay attention to all sensations in your body. For example, "Sitting the Mountain" takes you into a deep state of grounded awareness, in which your only goal is to become as fully conscious of the present moment as possible. *One-pointed* meditation is a type of mindfulness meditation, and is accomplished by focusing your attention on a single point such as your breath or a candle flame. It trains the mind to concentrate.

Clearing meditations have as their purpose the releasing of unwanted emotions, thoughts, or energies. Both "Tracing and Letting Go of Blocks" and "Unhooking" are clearing meditations that combine guided imagery and insight with the intention of clearing.

Many meditations are combinations of techniques. Any meditation that asks you to visualize something is a guided imagery meditation, such as "Self-Healing," in which you "see" your physical body moving from illness into health. Going into a memory to feel the emotions embodied there and gain new insight into them is a *sensory* meditation combined with an insight meditation. When these three strategies are combined, such as in "Finding Your Weak Link," you experience a memory of a situation through guided imagery; sensory awareness by the re-experiencing of emotions and how they affect your body; and new insight from examining the interconnections involved, which are sometimes pinpointed through carefully constructed questions introduced during the meditation.

Strengthening meditations are constructed to take you through a process of moving from an unwanted state of weakness or vulnerability to a state in which you can experience yourself as stronger, healthier, or more powerful. Many people in our culture are overwhelmed by the constant bombardment of other people, noise, traffic, pollution, and fast-moving visual images. "Strengthening Your Aura" is a Psychic Self-Defense meditation used for producing and reinforcing a feeling of clear and well-defined energetic boundaries, which can lead to an experience of calm and protection.

The Purpose of Meditation

The intention behind these meditation techniques is to bring you to an awareness of your inner life. The external world is not the only world that exists. No matter what religion you already practice, or spiritual path you follow, these meditations can help you reach a deeper place of healing within yourself. In the end, most religions and spiritual paths have a common goal: an awareness that attention to the life within you is essential, and that through awakening and touching this inner life, we can have a deeper and more meaningful connection with ourselves and our Creator. We can even find relief from suffering, and experience deep compassion and peace.

The meditations in this book have been divided into five sections: "Healing the Body," "Forgiveness," "Psychic Self-Defense," "Creating a New Life," and "Helping Others Heal." In the more than twenty years that I have been practicing the art and science of spiritual healing, these are the five topics that I have found to be the most important to people in their healing process. When our physical body is ill or in pain, we want immediate relief and permanent healing, if possible. This is why I have placed this chapter first. In the process of healing our bodies, however, we often discover that the deeper wounds of the heart are underlying our symptoms. When we are in conflict with people we love or care about, it can drain life force that is needed for healing. Through forgiveness, we can free this emotional energy so that it can participate in our physical healing. The next step is to make sure that we protect our healing process and the new energies that are being generated. When we are assaulted by a world filled with people, noise, pollution, crime, and horrifying news reports, it becomes difficult to keep the integrity of our own boundaries. A good analogy would be covering a wound with a bandage to protect it from germs and injury. Practicing Psychic Self-Defense keeps us protected from the negative energies around us so that we can heal as effectively as possible. In following these steps of healing, we often realize that we need to change direction, end our old ways of doing things, and create new lives for ourselves. "Creating a New Life" provides meditations that can help you do this. Once you have experienced the self-healing that these first four chapters have to offer, you may feel ready to offer comfort, care, compassion, and healing to loved ones or the people you work with on a professional basis. "Helping Others Heal" provides you with guided meditations and exercises that can be used for this purpose.

The meditations within each chapter have been arranged to provide you with the most benefit when they are done consecutively.

You may, of course, do them in whatever order you wish. I believe, however, that you will find each builds upon the one before it and, to achieve optimal healing, you may wish to do them in the order in which they are presented.

Each chapter contains a variety of meditation techniques: *relaxation, insight, clearing, strengthening,* and so on. You will have an opportunity to choose the topics that you feel will be most beneficial for you, as well as to notice how you respond to the different types of techniques. Each of the five chapters begins with an introduction, and each meditation has a brief description of its purpose and process.

If you are not used to meditating, it may be helpful to begin with "Deep Relaxation," doing this meditation once or twice a day for the first week. Read the meditation completely before beginning, then close your eyes and follow the process. If you have the audio tapes that coordinate with this book, all you need to do is to place the tape in a cassette player and turn it on. Close your eyes and my voice will guide you through the meditation.

The second week, you may wish to add a meditation of your choice or substitute the new meditation for the former one. If you are following in the order presented, the next meditation is "Opening the Chakras with White Light." It is advisable to try out a new meditation on a weekend or your day off, until you see how you respond to it. Some meditations may feel easy and comfortable, while others may feel difficult or painful. If, for instance, you wish to help heal your heart from the loss of a loved one by using "Dealing with Loss," you may find that this meditation is best done in the evening or on a weekend, when you have time to process your emotions.

The meditations that bring up strong emotions are often the most deeply healing, although people tend to avoid them at first. It is uncomfortable, even anxiety-producing, to feel an emotion that has been repressed. That is why we tend to push down into unconsciousness those feelings that we do not believe we can handle effectively or easily. If any of the meditations bring up painful feelings for you, it may be beneficial to seek guidance or counseling from someone who can offer you support. If you are already in psychotherapy, psychoanalysis, or counseling, you already have a safe container in which to explore these feelings. If you are close to your minister, priest, or rabbi, this person may be able to provide guidance as well. Sometimes all that is needed is a caring friend to listen. Whatever option you choose, it is important to seek out support for any painful or anxiety-producing feelings that may arise. As you do, you will begin to notice that these feelings are coming up and out so that you can heal them and integrate this healing into your life.

Practicing Meditation

The more you meditate, the easier it will become. You may find, like many people, that meditation can be pleasurable, relaxing, and deeply peaceful. Before you begin, you should choose a quiet place in your house or apartment that you can retreat to for meditation. Many people prefer to devote an entire room to this purpose, however, most of us choose the corner of a bedroom or study. A comfortable chair, cushion, or rug is all that is needed. You may wish to make this meditation corner more peaceful and spiritual by positioning a small table with a lit candle in front of you, and by playing some slow and pleasant music in the background. The candle can help you still your mind if you look at its flame for a few seconds before beginning. You also may wish to place a meaningful object on the table that makes you feel connected with your religion or spiritual path: a cross, Star of David, or a photo of a guru, for example. You may find, as many people do, that over time you will place additional objects on your table: a seashell from a walk along the beach, a robin's egg that you found, or a quartz crystal that someone gave you.

Once your meditation corner is set up, you need to choose a time of the day during which you will not be interrupted. Early morning, before everyone else is up and about, is often the best time. You can do "Self-Healing" for a physical condition or "Strengthening Your Aura" before going off to work.

The evening can also be a beneficial time. You may find that meditating right after you get home from work can help you release the tensions of the day. One of my students used to do "Unhooking" every day, so that she could release all the negative energies from people at work. If you have children, you may find that the best time is after they have gone to bed. Meditating in the evening or right before going to bed can produce a deeper and more peaceful sleep. If you have any trouble sleeping, you may find that "Deep Relaxation" or "Healing Affirmations" will help you drift off.

You may read any of the meditations in the first four chapters to a friend, family member, or patient. If you wish to do a simple hands-on healing with someone, you can refer to "Laying-on-of-Hands" in chapter 5. With the exception of "Distant Healing," you will find that these exercises and meditations are designed to be used with a minimum of two people. By simply reading the meditation aloud, you can provide a guided process that will stimulate intuitive sensitivities and healing energies in the practitioners.

When reading the meditations to another person, this individual should sit or lie down comfortably, uncross the arms and legs, and close the eyes. Your voice needs to be slow and soothing. Make sure to pause at the end of each paragraph for ten to twenty seconds to allow the person time to process the instruction or suggestion. Pause for five seconds at the end of each six dots . . . . . . within the paragraph. Until you get used to the rhythm of reading a meditation aloud, you should refer to a watch or clock for the timing. Most people unknowingly read too fast the first few times. What seems overly slow to the reader may feel just right to the listener.

The most important thing to remember about meditation is that it has the potential to awaken the healer within you and others. Healing meditations are valuable adjuncts to medical treatment.

Please do *not* use them in place of medical treatment. Meditating can help us heal physically, emotionally, mentally, and spiritually. All you have to do is pick a meditation, sit down, and close your eyes!

CHAPTER 1

Healing Your Body

Deep Relaxation

Opening the Chakras with White Light

Opening the Chakras with Color

Chakra Guides

Tracing and Letting Go of Blocks

Communicating with Your Body

Reclaiming Your Face

Reclaiming Your Body

Pain Relief

Healing Affirmations

Self-Healing

Color Healing

*W*e are all physical embodiments of Spirit. We are all creations of God. Most of us are born perfectly healthy and whole into an imperfect world. We are exposed to bacteria, viruses, pollution, and noise, as well as the stresses of work and family. Sometimes we have genes that give us tendencies to develop certain diseases. Given all these factors, we would like to know how to stay as healthy as possible, and how to recover from symptoms and illnesses, dis-eases, as we encounter them.

The meditations in this chapter will help you experience your body in new ways. Actually, you will find that you have more than one body. In addition to the configuration of cells that makes up your physical body, you also have an *etheric body*, or subtle energy body. This body is comprised of the life force, the energy field that keeps you alive. Scientists don't fully understand where this comes from or where it goes, but it is obvious to anyone with a spiritual orientation that we are more than just the sum of cells and chemicals. The cells and chemicals that comprise the body are still present when someone dies, but their "spirit" has left, as we say.

It is this spirit that lives within the temple of your body, and that can participate in its state of health. The etheric body consists of the *chakras,* or subtle energy centers. The word chakra comes from the Sanskrit for "wheel" and refers to the centers of light and subtle energies that we hold in our etheric body, our subtle energy body. *Kundalini* energy is the movement of these energies through our spine, our chakras, and the *nadis,* the internal channels on each side of our spine. The subtle energy body is invisible to most people, but it is this configuration of light energy that supplies our physical body with life force. It is the energetic substance of which we are composed. Subtle energies form the life field in and around the body. It is the *astral body,* or soul body, that, unlike the etheric body, can separate out from the physical body during sleep, surgery, or traumatic events, such as car accidents. People often report experiences of looking down at their own physical bodies during such occurrences.

The Hindus and Buddhists have used chakras for thousands of years in meditation and yogic practice. The chakras are centers of light energy, rising from the root chakra at the base of the spine, which is a denser, warmer, heavier vibration, and more connected to earth; to the crown chakra at the top of the head, which is a lighter, finer, faster frequency, and more connected to the heavens. Each chakra has a particular color, sound, quality, body area or organ, animal, food, gemstone, and planet associated with it. The colors range from red to violet, just as in the light spectrum. Here is a simple description of the seven major chakras, from my own work:

CHAKRA	COLOR	QUALITIES, ENERGIES	BODY LOCATION AFFECTED
1	red	survival, grounding, safety, security	coccyx bone, legs, knees, ankles, feet, skin, colon, bones
2	orange	sexuality, clairsentience, creative life force	pelvis, reproductive organs, lower back, bladder
3	yellow	physical willpower, motivation, vitality, instinct	digestion, stomach, liver, gall bladder, pancreas, spleen, middle spine, kidneys, adrenal glands, intestines
4	green	love, compassion, emotional empathy	heart, thymus gland, breasts, lungs, upper back, shoulders, arms, hands
5	blue	self-expression, clairaudience	throat, thyroid gland, neck, jaw, teeth, ears, sinuses
6	indigo	vision, psychic sight, clairvoyance, telepathy	third eye between eyebrows, pineal and pituitary glands, eyes

| 7 | violet | spiritual consciousness, direct knowing | crown of head, brain, scalp, hair |

When the chakras are open and balanced in relation to each other, they allow the free flow of subtle energies throughout the body. In Chinese acupuncture, now being accepted by Western medicine, there are energy meridians that connect all the organs, nerves, and muscles. They cannot be seen with the physical eyes, but their energies can be seen with the third eye. They are felt by taking a person's pulses, and noting the responses when acupuncture needles are placed at certain designated points. In much the same way, the energies of the chakras create an energy system throughout the subtle and physical bodies that can be felt with the hands and sensed intuitively. Although more centered through the torso than the meridians, which run vertically along the limbs as well as the torso, these spiraling wheels of energy have effects through all the muscles, nerves, and organs.

The chakras rotate in the center of the physical body, opening to the outside world through both the front and back. Sometimes the rotation is clockwise, sometimes counterclockwise. It is best to allow your chakras to choose their own direction. The first chakra, the center of survival, safety, and grounding, also opens straight down into the earth and connects us with it. The more I have worked with scanning the chakras, the more aware I have become of the energies at the back of the body holding both the energies of the past and the supporting energies of the body and soul. In fact, the past, including past lives, usually *is* the supporting energy of the body and soul. The energies moving in and out of the chakras through the front of the body are the forward-moving energies that keep us connected with the present and future, as well as the people and events in our lives now.

When a chakra is closed, shut down, or blocked in some way by a repressed emotion or memory, it can lead to physical symptoms. An obvious example to most people is that when we are afraid to express our feelings, sometimes our throat tightens up. The throat chakra is the center of self-expression and verbal creativity. We use the metaphor *broken-hearted* when speaking of the loss of love, and the heart chakra is the center of love. When the grief is enormous and prolonged, the heart chakra tends to become so overwhelmed with this pain that it can affect the physical heart and the intercostal muscles in the chest. An emergency-room physician, a former student of mine, told me that 80 percent of the people who come in thinking that they are having a heart attack actually have a condition called *costochondritis,* or inflammation of the intercostal muscles in the chest. Emotional stress has become so enormous for these people, and held within the heart chakra and chest, that it becomes a painful and frightening physical symptom.

When we deal with our emotions as they arise, rather than repress them down into our bodies, we can often prevent these physical symptoms. Immune system researchers Candace Pert and Margaret Kenemy have shown that we really do feel physically what we are feeling emotionally, and that by giving expression to these feelings, we increase the immune-system response in the body. The more science learns about the interconnections between the body, emotions, and thoughts, the more it finds itself agreeing with many of the mystical traditions of both East and West.

The chakras give us a way to work with both prevention and treatment of dis-ease by keeping them open and flowing with energy, such as in the meditations "Opening the Chakras with White Light" and "Opening the Chakras with Color." If you are just beginning to meditate with the chakras, using white light may be a simpler way to begin. Once you have become comfortable and facile with visualizing white light, using color is the next step. In doing these meditations, we also learn which chakras are open and which may be holding emotions and memories that we need to confront. Most people have two or three chakras that produce physical, emotional, mental, or spiritual symptoms. In "Tracing and Letting Go of Blocks," you can choose one of these chakras to focus on more deeply. By the end of this meditation you will have more insight into the ways that you are blocking your energy and emotions.

"Chakra Guides" also gives you a way to understand your chakras. This meditation is a favorite with children. It uses imaginary dialogues with animal guides or *allies* as they are called in shamanism, to give us ideas about the state of health and energy at each center. The entire meditation can be done by an adult, but most children under ten years of age will probably have enough attention span for only one, two, or three of the chakras at any one sitting.

If prevention is not possible, and there is a physical symptom, condition, or illness already present, you may wish to use "Communicating with Your Body." This meditation takes our ability to use a free-flowing imagination to identify with the condition and then dialogue with it, almost as though it had a mind of its own, which sometimes an illness seems to have! It is very important when using this dialoguing process to allow your imagination to flow freely. Don't judge the material that comes forth, and don't try to edit it, even if you get something that seems ridiculous. It may be a valuable insight when examined further. By the end of "Communicating with Your Body," you will probably have a better idea of how you can help yourself get well.

When I first created the meditations "Reclaiming Your Face" and "Reclaiming Your Body," I had a particular friend in mind. Her mother had tied her legs together when she was a toddler, and then tied her to the crib so she couldn't get out. She had a lot of anger and constriction in her legs. In doing the meditation, she was able to work through this memory, the emotions it elicited, and reclaim the energy and movement in her legs. Some people have similar issues in their face: features that they don't like or that remind them of their father or mother.

If you are experiencing physical pain, "Pain Relief" is a deeply relaxing and healing meditation. You may even find that you fall asleep during or shortly after the meditation. This added benefit is also true of "Color Healing," "Healing Affirmations," and "Self-Healing." Their intention is to direct the body into such a deeply peaceful state that the healing images and affirmations can begin to take effect and trigger the body's own healing responses. As we all know, the body is a miraculous self-healing organism. When we learn to speak its language through using the imagination, and remove both internal and external conflicts, we provide an opportunity for the brain and body to "re-member" the healing instructions already encoded by God.

Deep Relaxation

This meditation is a wonderful preliminary to use before any of the other meditations. It will help you relax physically and mentally, so that you can concentrate more deeply. It can also be used when you get home from work or before you go to sleep. If you are fully dressed, you may wish to take off your shoes and eyeglasses, and loosen your belt or tie. This meditation can be done sitting or lying down, in full or dimmed light, or even with the lights turned off. If you fall asleep in bed while doing the meditation, that's great!

Find a comfortable position, either sitting or lying down. Uncross your arms and legs, and close your eyes. Take a long, deep breath, and let it out slowly. Allow your breathing to become full, deep, and relaxed.

As you count from ten to zero, allow your rational mind to rest, and you will become more receptive to the wisdom of your soul and its healing power: ten—nine—eight—seven—six—five—four—three—two—one—zero. You are now very deeply relaxed.

Focus your attention on your toes. Get in touch with how your toes feel. Wiggle them. You may feel a slight tingling or flow of energy. Allow your toes to relax.

Allow this sensation of relaxation to gently move upward into your feet.

Feel the tops, bottoms, and sides of your feet flowing with the gentle sensation of relaxation.

Now gradually allow this sensation to move up into your ankles. Breathe.

Continue to allow the sensation of relaxation to move inch by inch into your calves.

As you allow the muscles in your calves to relax, you may feel a sensation of warmth as the blood flows smoothly and the nerves balance.

Gradually allow the sensation of relaxation to continue up into your knees.

Your lower legs are completely relaxed now.

You are very comfortable, and your breathing is becoming more and more deeply relaxed.

Allow the sensation of relaxation to move into your thighs.

And into your groin and hip areas.

Feel your pelvis, buttocks, and lower back becoming more and more relaxed. Breathe.

Your entire lower body is relaxed. All the muscles, nerves, and organs are in a deep state of relaxation.

Allow this sensation of deep relaxation to spread up into your stomach muscles, through your rib cage and middle back.

Breathe deeply as you feel your solar plexus open and relax.

Allow this sensation of relaxation to move up into your chest and heart, your lungs and upper back.

Feel your shoulders beginning to relax and the sensation spreading down your arms and into your hands and fingers.

Allow this sensation of relaxation to move up into your neck and jaw, mouth and face. Drop your jaw slightly.

You can feel relaxing all the muscles in your face and forehead, especially between your eyebrows.

Your mind is resting, and you can feel your scalp relaxing.

Your whole body is completely relaxed now, and your mind is still.

Take a moment to gently allow your awareness to scan through your body, and see if there are any areas that need to relax more deeply.

Breathe and let go into these areas, relaxing them even more deeply.

You may continue in this deep state of relaxation for as long as you wish. When you are ready to open your eyes, count up from one to ten: one–two–three–four–five–six–seven–eight–nine–ten.

Opening the Chakras with White Light

✤ *The chakras are the wheels of energy in our subtle body that contain and distribute life force. In opening these centers, we mobilize healing throughout our subtle energy body as well as our physical body. We also balance our emotional, mental, and spiritual levels of consciousness. Sometimes the chakras move clockwise, sometimes counterclockwise. Allow each chakra to find its natural flow.*

Find a comfortable position, either sitting or lying down. Uncross your arms and legs, and close your eyes. Take a long, deep breath, and let it out slowly. Allow your breathing to become full, deep, and relaxed.

As you count from ten to zero, allow your rational mind to rest, and you will become more receptive to the wisdom of your soul and its healing power: ten–nine–eight–seven–six–five–four–three–two–one–zero. You are now very deeply relaxed.

Focus your attention far above the top of your head, out into the heavens, and get in touch with a brilliant, powerful, white light and energy flowing down toward you.

Allow yourself to experience this light energy flowing all around you and through you, filling your body with its radiance. With each breath, you inhale this light. As it fills and surrounds you, it gently permeates your entire being and joins the river of life energy already filling your body.

Focus your attention at the base of your spine, where your coccyx bone is located. This is your root chakra, your center of security, safety, and grounding in the physical world. Get in touch with the white light in your first chakra as it gently moves in a circular motion.

Feel this white light as energy flowing down through your legs and feet and into the ground, connecting you with Mother Earth.

Notice any sensations and emotions that arise as you connect with the physical nature of your body and Mother Earth.

Allow the energy in your first chakra to gradually continue flowing upward in a spiral motion into your second chakra, in the center of your pelvis.

This is your center of sexuality and creative life force. As the light energy opens your second chakra, it moves gently in a circular motion.

Notice any sensations and emotions that arise as you connect with your sexuality and creative life force.

Now gradually allow the energy in your second chakra to continue flowing upward in a spiral motion into your third chakra, at your solar plexus in the center of your rib cage.

This is your center of physical willpower, motivation, and vitality. As the light energy opens your third chakra, it moves gently in a circular motion.

Notice any sensations and emotions that arise as you connect with your physical willpower, motivation, and vitality.

Now gradually allow the energy in your third chakra to continue flowing upward in a spiral motion into your fourth chakra, your heart center in the middle of your chest.

This is your center of love and compassion. As the light energy opens your fourth chakra, it moves gently in a circular motion.

Notice any sensations and emotions that arise as you connect with your heart.

Now gradually allow the energy in your heart chakra to continue flowing upward in a spiral motion into your fifth chakra, in the center of your throat.

This is your center of self-expression. As the light energy opens your fifth chakra, it moves gently in a circular motion.

Notice any sensations and emotions that arise as you connect with your self-expression.

Now gradually allow the energy in your fifth chakra to continue flowing upward in a spiral motion into your sixth chakra, between your eyebrows.

This is your center of psychic sight and true vision. As the light energy opens your third eye, it moves gently in a circular motion.

Notice any sensations and emotions that arise as you connect with your ability to see clearly.

Now gradually allow the energy in your third eye to continue flowing upward in a spiral motion into your seventh chakra, at the crown of your head.

This is your center of spiritual consciousness and direct knowing. As the light energy opens your seventh chakra, it moves gently in a circular motion.

Notice any sensations and emotions that arise as you connect with your spiritual consciousness.

Now allow your awareness to slowly scan down through all of your chakras. Allow yourself to feel the energy slowly moving in a circular motion in each center.

When you reach your first chakra at the base of your spine, reconnect with the light energy moving down through your legs and feet to give you a feeling of grounding.

On the count of ten, you may open your eyes: one–two–three–four–five–six–seven–eight–nine–ten. Give yourself a minute or two to become accustomed to being back in the room with your eyes open.

Opening the Chakras with Color

✤ *This meditation is the same as the previous exercise with one difference: It guides you in visualizing a color at each chakra. Visualizing color will help you open your third eye, your center of psychic sight and clear vision. Light energy runs the red-to-violet spectrum, and so do the chakras. The first chakra at the base of the spine, security, has the slower, denser, warmer vibration of red light; whereas the seventh chakra at the crown of the head, spiritual consciousness, has the faster, lighter, cooler vibration of violet. Allow yourself to feel the difference as your awareness shifts through all seven chakras.*

Find a comfortable position, either sitting or lying down. Uncross your arms and legs, and close your eyes. Take a long, deep breath, and let it out slowly. Allow your breathing to become full, deep, and relaxed.

As you count from ten to zero, allow your rational mind to rest, and you will become more receptive to the wisdom of your soul and its healing power: ten–nine–eight–seven–six–five–four–three–two–one–zero. You are now very deeply relaxed.

Focus your attention far above the top of your head, out into the heavens, and get in touch with a brilliant, powerful, white light and energy flowing down toward you.

Allow yourself to experience this light energy flowing all around you and through you, filling your body with its radiance. With each breath, you inhale this light. As it fills and surrounds you, it gently permeates your entire being and joins the river of life energy already filling your body.

Focus your attention at the base of your spine, where your coccyx bone is located. This is your root chakra, your center of security, safety, and grounding in the physical world. Get in touch with the white light in your first chakra as it gently moves in a circular motion.

As the light energy slowly opens your root chakra, it becomes a bright red. Feel the energy and vibration of this red light as it gently moves in a circular motion.

Feel this red light energy flowing down through your legs and feet and into the ground, connecting you with Mother Earth.

Notice any sensations and emotions that arise as you connect with the physical nature of your body and Mother Earth.

Now gradually allow the energy in your first chakra to continue flowing upward in a spiral motion into your second chakra, in the center of your pelvis.

This is your center of sexuality and creative life force. As the light energy opens your second chakra, it becomes a bright orange and moves gently in a circular motion.

Notice any sensations and emotions that arise as you connect with your sexuality and creative life force.

Now gradually allow the energy in your second chakra to continue flowing upward in a spiral motion into your third chakra, at your solar plexus between your rib cage.

This is your center of physical willpower, motivation, and vitality. As the light energy opens your third chakra, it becomes a bright yellow and moves gently in a circular motion.

Notice any sensations and emotions that arise as you connect with your physical willpower, motivation, and vitality.

Now gradually allow the energy in your third chakra to continue flowing upward in a spiral motion into your fourth chakra, your heart center in the middle of your chest.

This is your center of love and compassion. As the light energy opens your fourth chakra, it becomes a bright green and moves gently in a circular motion.

Notice any sensations and emotions that arise as you connect with your heart.

Now gradually allow the energy in your heart chakra to continue flowing upward in a spiral motion into your fifth chakra in the center of your throat.

This is your center of self-expression. As the light energy opens your fifth chakra, it becomes a bright blue and moves gently in a circular motion.

Notice any sensations and emotions that arise as you connect with your self-expression.

Now gradually allow the energy in your fifth chakra to continue flowing upward in a spiral motion into your sixth chakra, between your eyebrows.

This is your center of psychic sight and true vision. As the light energy opens your third eye, it becomes a bright indigo or lapis (blue-purple) and moves gently in a circular motion.

Notice any sensations and emotions that arise as you connect with your ability to see clearly.

Now gradually allow the energy in your third eye to continue flowing upward in a spiral motion into your seventh chakra, at the crown of your head.

This is your center of spiritual consciousness and direct knowing. As the light energy opens your seventh chakra, it becomes a bright violet and moves gently in a circular motion.

Notice any sensations and emotions that arise as you connect with your spiritual consciousness.

Now allow your awareness to slowly scan down through all of your chakras. As you see each color, allow yourself to feel the energy slowly moving in a circular motion in each center.

When you reach your first chakra, at the base of your spine, reconnect with the red light energy moving down through your legs and feet as it gives you a feeling of grounding.

On the count of ten, you may open your eyes: one–two–three–four–five–six–seven–eight–nine–ten. Give yourself a minute or two to become accustomed to being back in the room with your eyes open.

Chakra Guides

❧ *Make sure you have done one of the "Opening the Chakras" meditations before you attempt this one, so that you feel comfortable in knowing where your chakras are located and how to access them. You want to allow your imagination free play as you become conscious of each chakra and the animal guide or ally that you will find there. Sometimes the animals will talk to you in words, but they may also talk through movement, expression, or action. This meditation can be fun, as well as insightful. It is very important that you take what you get— don't judge and don't edit! If you get an animal that you don't like, don't change it! Sometimes the things we don't like have much to teach us.*

Find a comfortable position, either sitting or lying down. Uncross your arms and legs, and close your eyes. Take a long, deep breath, and let it out slowly. Allow your breathing to become full, deep, and relaxed.

As you count from ten to zero, allow your rational mind to rest, and you will become more receptive to the wisdom of your soul and its healing power: ten—nine—eight—seven—six—five—four—three—two—one—zero. You are now very deeply relaxed.

Focus your attention far above the top of your head, out into the heavens, and get in touch with a brilliant, powerful, white light and energy flowing down toward you.

Allow yourself to experience this light energy flowing all around you and through you, filling your body with its radiance. With each breath, you inhale this light. As it fills and surrounds you, it gently permeates your entire being and joins the river of life energy already filling your body.

Focus your attention at the base of your spine, where your coccyx bone is located. This is your root chakra, your center of security, safety, and grounding in the physical world. Get in touch with the white light in your first chakra as it gently moves in a circular motion.

Feel this white light as energy flowing down through your legs and feet and into the ground, connecting you with Mother Earth.

On the count of three you will see an animal guide in your first chakra: one–two–three. Ask it its name. Ask this guide if there is anything you are blocking or holding onto in this center, and pay careful attention to its response.

Ask your guide how it can help you to open the energy at this center.

Express your gratitude to this guide, and bid farewell.

Now gradually allow the energy in your first chakra to continue flowing upward in a spiral motion into your second chakra, in the center of your pelvis.

This is your center of sexuality and creative life force. As the light energy opens your second chakra, it moves gently in a circular motion.

On the count of three you will see an animal guide in this chakra: one–two–three. Ask it its name. Ask this guide if there is anything you are blocking or holding onto in this center, and pay careful attention to its response.

Ask your guide how it can help you to open the energy at this center.

Express your gratitude to this guide, and bid farewell.

Now gradually allow the energy in your second chakra to continue flowing upward in a spiral motion into your third chakra, at your solar plexus in the center of your rib cage.

This is your center of physical willpower, motivation, and vitality. As the light energy opens your third chakra, it moves gently in a circular motion.

On the count of three you will see an animal guide in this chakra: one–two–three. Ask it its name. Ask this guide if there is anything you are blocking or holding onto in this center, and pay careful attention to its response.

Ask your guide how it can help you to open the energy at this center.

Express your gratitude to this guide, and bid farewell.

Now gradually allow the energy in your third chakra to continue flowing upward in a spiral motion into your fourth chakra, your heart center in the middle of your chest.

This is your center of love and compassion. As the light energy opens your fourth chakra, it moves gently in a circular motion.

On the count of three you will see an animal guide in this chakra: one–two–three. Ask it its name. Ask this guide if there is anything you are blocking or holding onto in this center, and pay careful attention to its response.

Ask your guide how it can help you to open the energy at this center.

Express your gratitude to this guide, and bid farewell.

Now gradually allow the energy in your heart chakra to continue flowing upward in a spiral motion into your fifth chakra, in the center of your throat.

This is your center of self-expression. As the light energy opens your fifth chakra, it moves gently in a circular motion.

On the count of three you will see an animal guide in this chakra: one–two–three. Ask it it's name. Ask this guide if there is anything you are blocking or holding onto in this center, and pay careful attention to its response.

Ask your guide how it can help you to open the energy at this center.

Express your gratitude to this guide, and bid farewell.

Now gradually allow the energy in your fifth chakra to continue flowing upward in a spiral motion into your sixth chakra, between your eyebrows.

This is your center of psychic sight and true vision. As the light energy opens your third eye, it moves gently in a circular motion.

On the count of three you will see an animal guide in this chakra: one–two–three. Ask it its name. Ask this guide if there is anything you are blocking or holding onto in this center, and pay careful attention to its response.

Ask your guide how it can help you to open the energy at this center.

Express your gratitude to this guide, and bid farewell.

Now gradually allow the energy in your third eye to continue flowing upward in a spiral motion into your seventh chakra, at the crown of your head.

This is your center of spiritual consciousness and direct knowing. As the light energy opens your seventh chakra, it moves gently in a circular motion.

On the count of three you will see an animal guide in this chakra: one–two–three. Ask it its name. Ask this guide if there is anything you are blocking or holding onto in this center, and pay careful attention to its response.

Ask your guide how it can help you to open the energy at this center.

Express your gratitude to this guide, and bid farewell.

Now allow your awareness to slowly scan down through all your chakras and their guides. Allow yourself to feel the energy slowly moving in a circular motion in each center.

When you reach your first chakra, at the base of your spine, re-connect with the light energy moving down through your legs and feet to give you a feeling of grounding.

On the count of ten, you may open your eyes: one–two–three–four–five–six–seven–eight–nine–ten. Give yourself a minute or two to become accustomed to being back in the room with your eyes open.

Tracing and Letting Go of Blocks

✥ *After doing the previous meditations, you should have a pretty good idea of which chakras are troublesome for you. Certain chakras may give you physical discomfort when you become aware of them, or an unpleasant emotion may arise. Your animal guides may have called your attention to certain energy blockages. Or you may feel or see nothing at all when you try to become conscious of a few chakras. This meditation will allow you to choose one of these chakras to focus on more deeply, with the intention of understanding it better and allowing the energy to flow more freely at this location.*

Find a comfortable position, either sitting or lying down. Uncross your arms and legs, and close your eyes. Take a long, deep breath, and let it out slowly. Allow your breathing to become full, deep, and relaxed.

As you count from ten to zero, allow your rational mind to rest, and you will become more receptive to the wisdom of your soul and its healing power: ten—nine—eight—seven—six—five—four—three—two—one—zero. You are now very deeply relaxed.

Focus your attention far above the top of your head, out into the heavens, and get in touch with a brilliant, powerful, white light and energy flowing down toward you.

Allow yourself to experience this light energy flowing all around you and through you, filling your body with its radiance. With each breath, you inhale this light. As it fills and surrounds you, it gently permeates your entire being and joins the river of life energy already filling your body.

Take a long, deep breath and focus your attention on the chakra you wish to explore. Allow the white light and energy flowing through your body to move into this area.

What sensations are you experiencing in this chakra?

What sensations are you feeling in this part of yourself?

Allow the answers to come easily and spontaneously from your unconscious.

What sensations are you experiencing in this part of your body?

What memories do you associate with these sensations?

What memories do you associate with this part of your body?

What memories are connected with this chakra? Breathe.

Are you feeling any emotions as you connect with these memories?

Allow yourself to experience any emotions that you may be holding in this part of your body.

What emotions are connected with this chakra?

Have you made any judgments associated with these emotions and memories?

What judgments have you made about yourself and your life?

What judgments have you made about others?

What decisions have you made from these judgments, memories, and emotions?

What actions have you taken based on these decisions?

Now take a long, deep breath and become aware of how you are holding or blocking your energy in this chakra.

What would you need to let go of in order to open the energy here?

What would you need to feel, experience, or change?

Are you willing to open the energy here?

If you are, then image yourself making these changes and letting go in some way.

Allow yourself to feel, in your body, a release of energy, a letting go on physical, emotional, and mental levels. Breathe.

Staying in touch with how you feel now, you may open your eyes on the count of ten: one–two–three–four–five–six–seven–eight–nine–ten.

Communicating with Your Body

✤ *This meditation will assist you in using the wisdom of your soul to gain new insights into the nature of a physical symptom or illness, and to understand some of what is needed for healing to take place. Before beginning this meditation, choose the physical symptom, illness, or location in your body on which you would like to focus.*

Find a comfortable position, either sitting or lying down. Uncross your arms and legs, and close your eyes. Take a long, deep breath, and let it out slowly. Allow your breathing to become full, deep, and relaxed.

As you count from ten to zero, allow your rational mind to rest, and you will become more receptive to the wisdom of your soul and its healing power: ten–nine–eight–seven–six–five–four–three–two–one–zero. You are now very deeply relaxed.

Focus your attention on a symptom or illness that you would like to understand, communicate with, and heal. Get in touch with all the sensations in this area of your body.

Allow yourself to remember any sensations you have experienced previously.

Now temporarily increase the intensity of these sensations.

Notice how you are doing this. Is there anything you are thinking or feeling that is increasing these sensations?

Now take a deep breath and release it. As you do, allow yourself to decrease the sensations.

Notice how you are doing this. Is there anything you are doing that is allowing you to relieve the sensations?

Now use your imagination and become the symptom or illness. Imagine being a child who is pretending to identify with the symptom or illness. What are you like? What personality do you have?

What is your life like?

What do you do to this person whose body you are in?

What are you trying to tell this person? What message are you trying to convey?

How have you changed this person's life?

How have you changed their relationships?

What emotions have you provoked?

Do you express something that this person cannot?

Is there something you help this person avoid?

Is there something you do for them? Are you useful in some way?

Are you protecting this person from anything or anyone?

What can this person do to heal you?

Now become yourself again. Tell the symptom or illness how you feel about what it has told you.

What feelings are you in touch with that you were not aware of before you developed this condition?

What needs and desires are you now in touch with?

Is there anything in your life that you want to change as a result of this condition?

Now picture your life beginning to change in the ways that you desire. Visualize yourself incorporating whatever you need for healing to take place.

See yourself as whole, healed, and filled with self-love.

On the count of ten you may open your eyes: one–two–three–four–five–six–seven–eight–nine–ten.

Reclaiming Your Face

✥ *This meditation will allow you to explore your face, and to get in touch with an area or feature with which you are not comfortable. In doing so, you may find that a particular feature reminds you of someone. You have the opportunity to reclaim this part of your face as your own.*

Find a comfortable position, either sitting or lying down. Uncross your arms and legs, and close your eyes. Take a long, deep breath, and let it out slowly. Allow your breathing to become full, deep, and relaxed.

As you count from ten to zero, allow your rational mind to rest, and you will become more receptive to the wisdom of your soul and its healing power: ten–nine–eight–seven–six–five–four–three–two–one–zero. You are now very deeply relaxed.

Focus all your attention on your face. Get in touch with how your face feels.

Feel the muscles, bones, skin.

Feel the structure of your face.

Pay attention to any sensations you feel.

Focus your attention on each area of your face and each feature, separately.

Forehead.

Eyes.

Nose.

Mouth.

Jaw.

Chin.

Cheeks.

Ears.

Which areas can you feel strongly and distinctly?

Which areas do you feel only vaguely?

Which areas of your face feel tight or uncomfortable?

Which feature or area of your face do you like least or feel least connected with?

Focus all your attention on this area or feature. What do you notice?

What sensations do you feel?

How does this feature or area feel in relationship to the rest of your face?

Does it want to move in any way?

Switch roles and imagine yourself as this part of your face.

What are you like?

What is your life like?

What do you express about yourself?

What feelings do you express toward the rest of the world?

Now switch roles and become yourself again.

On the count of three, you will see the face or hear the name of the person you associate with this part of your face: one–two–three.

Notice how you feel as you realize who it is.

How does this person relate to this part of your face?

Is there some way in which they own this part?

Imagine this person standing in front of you, and tell them how you feel about their relationship to your face.

If you wish, imagine yourself releasing or giving back to this person any associations that you no longer want.

Now release this person's image. Visualize what you want this part of your face to express.

Image, as well as feel, this area of your face expressing exactly what you wish.

Hold this image in your mind clearly, and feel it strongly in your face.

Now feel this feature or area relating to the rest of your face in a new way.

Feel your entire face as whole, integrated, and expressive of your true feelings.

Staying in touch with this new sense of your face and the feelings that go with it, you may open your eyes on the count of ten: one–two–three–four–five–six–seven–eight–nine–ten.

Reclaiming Your Body

❧ *This meditation will allow you to explore your body, and to get in touch with an area or feature with which you are not comfortable. As with "Reclaiming Your Face," you may find that a particular feature reminds you of someone. You have the opportunity to reclaim this part of your body as your own.*

Find a comfortable position, either sitting or lying down. Uncross your arms and legs, and close your eyes. Take a long, deep breath, and let it out slowly. Allow your breathing to become full, deep, and relaxed.

As you count from ten to zero, allow your rational mind to rest, and you will become more receptive to the wisdom of your soul and its healing power: ten–nine–eight–seven–six–five–four–three–two–one–zero. You are now very deeply relaxed.

Focus all your attention on your body. Get in touch with how your body feels.

Feel the muscles, bones, and skin.

Feel the structure of your body.

Pay attention to any sensations you feel.

Focus your attention on each area of your body separately: feet and legs.

Hips, pelvis, and lower back.

Buttocks, groin, and genitals.

Torso, chest, and spine.

Shoulders, arms, and hands.

Neck and head.

Which areas can you feel strongly and distinctly?

Which areas do you feel only vaguely?

Which areas of your body feel tight or uncomfortable?

Which part of your body do you like least, or feel least connected with?

Focus all your attention on this area. What do you notice?

What sensations do you feel?

How does this part feel in relationship to the rest of your body?

Does it want to move in any way?

Switch roles and imagine yourself as this part of your body.

What are you like?

What is your life like?

What do you express about yourself?

What feelings do you express toward the rest of the world?

Now switch roles and become yourself again.

On the count of three, you will see the face or hear the name of the person you associate with this part of your body: one–two–three.

Notice how you feel as you realize who it is.

How does this person relate to this part of your body?

Is there some way that they own this part?

Imagine this person standing in front of you, and tell them how you feel about their relationship to your body.

If you wish, imagine yourself releasing or giving back to this person any associations that you no longer want.

Now release this person's image. Visualize what you want this part of your body to express.

Image, as well as feel, this part of your body expressing exactly what you wish.

Hold this image in your mind clearly, and feel it strongly in your body.

Now feel this feature or area relating to the rest of your body in a new way.

Feel your entire body as whole, integrated, and expressive of your true feelings.

Staying in touch with this new sense of your body and the feelings that go with it, you may open your eyes on the count of ten: one–two–three–four–five–six–seven–eight–nine–ten.

Pain Relief

✤ *This meditation will assist you in releasing physical pain, and place you in a deeply relaxed state. The most effective position is lying down, so that you can allow yourself to fall asleep at the end of the meditation.*

Find a comfortable position, either sitting or lying down. Uncross your arms and legs, and close your eyes. Take a long, deep breath, and let it out slowly. Allow your breathing to become full, deep, and relaxed.

As you count from ten to zero, allow your rational mind to rest, and you will become more receptive to the wisdom of your soul and its healing power: ten–nine–eight–seven–six–five–four–three–two–one–zero. You are now very deeply relaxed.

Focus your attention on the location in your body where you experience pain. Allow yourself to become aware of all the characteristics of this pain.

Is it sharp or dull? Hot or cold? Do you feel throbbing or pressure?

Are there any other characteristics?

How large or small is the pain? Over what area does it extend?

What shape is it? Allow yourself to feel it as three dimensional, with depth and height, width and volume.

What color is the pain?

Now allow yourself to temporarily increase the characteristics of the pain.

Notice how you are doing this. Is there anything you are thinking or feeling that is increasing the pain?

Now take a long, deep breath and release it. As you do, allow the pain to decrease.

Notice how you are doing this.

Now use your imagination and place yourself inside the center of the pain. What are you like?

What is your life like?

What are you trying to say? What message are you trying to convey?

Now begin to change your size, shape, and color in any way you wish.

What are you like now? What color? Shape? Size?

Now become yourself again. Visualize the pain projected out onto a movie screen.

What do you see? What color is it? Shape? Size? What is it doing?

Visualize it as changing color, shape, and size again. Watch it like a movie.

Visualize the screen as moving farther and farther away from you.

As you are watching the screen disappear, feel a cool blue light surrounding your body and head.

With each breath in you are taking in more of this cool blue light. Your entire body fills with its gentle presence and produces a deep state of relaxation.

Every cell in your body is filling with this gentle, cool blue light.

Cooling, comforting, healing, flowing throughout your entire body. You rest in a deep peace.

You may wish to remain in this deeply peaceful and healing place. You may even wish to drift into sleep.

Completely comfortable, relaxed, and healed.

Remaining in this state as long as you wish, you may open your eyes whenever you feel ready to count from one to ten: one–two–three–four–five–six–seven–eight–nine–ten.

Healing Affirmations

✤ *This meditation combines guided imagery with positive healing statements called* affirmations. *The right side of the brain produces images and the left side produces rational, linear statements. By combining the energies from both sides of the brain, you are strongly stimulating the healing potential within you.*

Find a comfortable position, either sitting or lying down. Uncross your arms and legs, and close your eyes. Take a long, deep breath, and let it out slowly. Allow your breathing to become full, deep, and relaxed.

As you count from ten to zero, allow your rational mind to rest, and you will become more receptive to the wisdom of your soul and its healing power: ten–nine–eight–seven–six–five–four–three–two–one–zero. You are now very deeply relaxed.

Focus your attention far above the top of your head, out into the heavens, and get in touch with a brilliant, powerful, white light and energy flowing down toward you.

Allow yourself to experience this light energy flowing all around you and through you, filling your body with its radiance.

With each breath, you inhale this light. As it fills and surrounds you, it gently permeates your entire being, and joins the river of life energy already flowing through your body.

Experience yourself dropping more and more deeply into a state of peace, harmony, and healing.

Allow yourself to experience the following affirmations as your own. If you are alone, you may repeat them out loud. Breathe.

My body is a universe unto itself.

My body is a universe unto itself.

My blood is the ocean of my universe. It washes clean my inner tissues, and brings nutrients and life to my body.

My blood is the ocean of my universe. It washes clean my inner tissues, and brings nutrients and life to my body.

My nerve energy is like the sun, empowering my body.

My nerve energy is like the sun, empowering my body.

My brain is the creative center of my universe. It gives signals of healing to all parts of my body.

My brain is the creative center of my universe. It gives signals of healing to all parts of my body.

All my organs are working in harmony, as Mother Nature creates balance in my body.

All my organs are working in harmony, as Mother Nature creates balance in my body.

Breathe.

Allow yourself to feel the truth of these affirmations.

Everything my body needs is being supplied.

Everything my body needs is being supplied.

I accept the healing taking place in me now.

I accept the healing taking place in me now.

I trust in the Higher Intelligence that permeates all Life to heal and strengthen me.

I trust in the Higher Intelligence that permeates all Life to heal and strengthen me.

Allow yourself to really feel and experience the healing that is taking place in you now.

I accept this healing.

I accept this healing.

Feel yourself glowing with white light and healing energy.

Knowing that this healing continues to take place in both visible and invisible ways, you may open your eyes on the count of ten: one–two–three–four–five–six–seven–eight–nine–ten.

Self-Healing

✣ *This meditation will assist you in focusing healing intention on a symptom, illness, or area of your body. By connecting your awareness, brain, and physical body through guided imagery, you are creating an opportunity for messages of healing to be sent where they are needed most. The immune system can respond to healing imagery.*

Find a comfortable position, either sitting or lying down. Uncross your arms and legs, and close your eyes. Take a long, deep breath, and let it out slowly. Allow your breathing to become full, deep, and relaxed.

As you count from ten to zero, allow your rational mind to rest, and you will become more receptive to the wisdom of your soul and its healing power: ten–nine–eight–seven–six–five–four–three–two–one–zero. You are now very deeply relaxed.

Focus your attention far above the top of your head, out into the heavens, and get in touch with a brilliant, powerful white light and energy flowing down toward you.

Allow yourself to experience this light energy flowing all around you and through you, filling your body with its radiance. With each breath, you inhale this light. As it fills and surrounds you, it gently permeates your entire being and joins the river of life energy already flowing through your body.

Focus your attention on the area of your body that needs healing. Breathe deeply and let go.

Allow yourself to feel and image the white light energy gently circulating through this area of your body. Light energy is the energy of Creation, reminding your body of its power to create healing and new life.

Image your blood circulation cleansing your tissues as it removes toxins and unwanted cells.

See and feel your bright red blood bringing new oxygen and nourishment to your tissues and bones.

Feel and visualize your nerves beginning to balance, relax, and send messages of healing throughout your body. Breathe.

Allow your body to harmonize all its healing energies while strengthening your immune system, muscles, nerves, organs, and bones.

See and feel this area of your body healing.

On the count of three, see your body as being totally and completely healed, and hold this image: one–two–three.

Imagine your body functioning exactly as you wish, and while holding this image of healing, repeat the following affirmation three times:

I accept my healing, and acknowledge the light within me.

I accept my healing, and acknowledge the light within me.

I accept my healing, and acknowledge the light within me.

Feel and see yourself in a complete state of healing. Breathe.

See your body and your whole being as healed, joyous, and radiant with light.

See yourself doing all the things you love to do and have always wanted to do.

Feel yourself radiant with healing energy and light, love, and joy.

Experience your true nature as healthy and whole.

On the count of three, you will receive a symbol of healing: one–two–three.

Breathe. Accept this symbol of healing. Visualize it in the area of your body that is now healing, and trust that it will continue to generate healing energy and new life.

Allow the meaning of this symbol to be a mystery, knowing that at some point you will understand its importance. Feel its presence within you, and experience it radiating light and healing.

You may open your eyes on the count of ten: one–two–three–four–five–six–seven–eight–nine–ten.

Color Healing

❖ *This meditation is similar to "Self-Healing," but uses the power of color to heal. Cool colors like violet, blue, and green, can be imaged for pain relief, and to reduce inflammation and infection. Warm colors like red, orange, and yellow, can be used to warm the body, produce relaxation, and increase blood flow. You can also pick a color that corresponds to the chakra closest to your physical symptom, as long as its effect is appropriate. For example, if you have a sore throat, you would pick the color blue, sky blue, because it is both the color of the throat chakra, as well as the color that cools inflammation and produces pain relief. If you choose a color and it doesn't feel right, or another color spontaneously comes to you during the meditation, allow yourself to use the new color.*

Find a comfortable position, either sitting or lying down. Uncross your arms and legs, and close your eyes. Take a long, deep breath, and let it out slowly. Allow your breathing to become full, deep, and relaxed.

As you count from ten to zero, allow your rational mind to rest, and you will become more receptive to the wisdom of your soul and its healing power: ten—nine—eight—seven—six—five—four—three—two—one—zero. You are now very deeply relaxed.

Focus your attention far above the top of your head, out into the heavens, and get in touch with the color of light and energy that you need for healing. Allow this light energy to flow down toward you.

Allow yourself to experience this light energy flowing all around you and through you, filling your body with its radiance. With each breath you inhale this healing color. As it fills and surrounds you, it gently permeates your entire being and joins the river of life energy already flowing through your body.

Focus your attention on the area of your body that needs healing. Breathe deeply and let go.

Allow yourself to feel and image this color of light energy gently circulating through this area of your body. Light energy is the energy of Creation, reminding your body of its power to create healing and new life.

Image your blood circulation cleansing your tissues as it removes toxins and unwanted cells.

See and feel your bright red blood bringing new oxygen and nourishment to your tissues and bones.

Feel and visualize your nerves beginning to balance, relax, and send messages of healing throughout your body. Breathe.

Allow your body to harmonize all its healing energies while strengthening your immune system, muscles, nerves, organs, and bones.

See and feel this area of your body healing.

On the count of three, see your body as being totally and completely healed, and hold this image: one–two–three.

Imagine your body functioning exactly as you wish, and while holding this image of healing, repeat the following affirmation three times.

I accept my healing, and acknowledge the light within me. Breathe.

I accept my healing, and acknowledge the light within me.

I accept my healing, and acknowledge the light within me.

Feel and see yourself in a complete state of healing.

See your body and your whole being as healed, joyous, and radiant with light.

See yourself doing all the things you love to do and have always wanted to do.

Feel yourself radiant with healing energy and light, love, and joy.

Experience your true nature as healthy and whole.

On the count of three, you will receive a symbol of healing: one–two–three.

Breathe. Accept this symbol of healing. Visualize this symbol in the area of your body that is now healing, and trust that it will continue to generate healing energy and new life.

Allow the meaning of this symbol to be a mystery, knowing that at some point you will understand its importance. Feel its presence within you and experience it radiating light and healing.

You may open your eyes on the count of ten: one–two–three–four–five–six–seven–eight–nine–ten.

CHAPTER 2

Forgiveness

*L*ove is the most powerful healing energy. We all have felt the enormous joy and gratitude that fills our hearts when we look into the eyes of someone we love or into the face of a newborn baby, and when we are in the deep peace of prayer with God.

The only thing that stands in the way of love is a lack of forgiveness. If we examine our relationships, we most likely will find the emotions of resentment, guilt, anger, fear, rage, anxiety, expectation, and disappointment. These emotions cloud how we feel about people, and sometimes become almost the totality of how we feel about them. During twenty years as a healer, I have noticed that what concerns people most, after their own physical health, is the health of their relationships. Feeling anger and resentment toward someone we want to love is painful.

We feel tremendous conflict in relationships. We may love and hate someone at the same time. We may wish them well, and a few hours later wish they would fall off the planet. Such conflict distresses the mind, breaks the heart, and creates havoc in the body. When our minds and hearts are in conflict, the natural and healthy balance of the body is thrown into chemical confusion. For example, if you are having an argument with your spouse or a friend, your adrenal glands are most likely pumping adrenaline, which makes you feel hot and agitated, preparing you to fight or flee. Your mind may be telling you that it is time to get out of this relationship *now,* but your heart may be begging you to stay. Your poor body is getting mixed signals and doesn't know what to do. It keeps pumping out more and more adrenaline, waiting for you to make a decision. In the meantime, your mixed feelings of anger and love leave you paralyzed.

Later that day, when you are at work, you may replay the argument over and over in your mind. Each time, the imagery process is creating signals from your brain down through your central nervous system and into your muscles and organs. Your shoulders and neck become tense. Your jaw clenches. Your stomach knots up and secretes more acid. Before you know it you have a headache and a stomachache. Your body is reliving the argument dozens of times.

Most people then reach for painkillers for the headache and an antacid for the stomachache. These only work temporarily because they only address the symptoms. The cause is the reliving of the argument—the lack of resolution of the situation and the participating emotions. If you never resolve the anger and resentment, but live with it for years, you will most likely wind up taking many painkillers and gallons of antacid. Over long periods of time, these synthetic chemicals can wreak havoc on your liver, kidneys, and stomach.

The only way off this endless treadmill is to resolve the situation and the emotions that are leading to the physical symptoms. Resolving your emotional responses means doing inner healing work. The external situation may be triggering your internal emotions, but most likely it is not the cause. The cause may be much deeper: someone or something that caused you to feel this way before. Maybe your parents fought a lot, or possibly there was a great deal of unspoken anger and resentment in your household. Whatever the scenario, sometimes the way we feel and respond in the present is a repetition of the way that we felt and responded in the past.

Using meditation techniques to deal with these past and present feelings is very effective, because it goes right to the origin of the pain rather than masking it. By looking inside ourselves and tracing our emotional responses back to when we first learned them, we can discover exactly what we are feeling. Doing this kind of deep, intensely concentrated work takes spiritual and emotional endurance, as well as a good sense of physical embodiment and grounding. It is like building muscles in a gym. We begin slowly, knowing that our muscles must get used to being exercised in order for them to accept the training. If we push ourselves too far, too fast, we may tear or injure our muscles. Then we may become afraid and tired, and do not want to continue. It is the same with emotional insight and mindfulness meditation. We must begin slowly and build endurance, such as with the meditation "Sitting the Mountain." The purpose of this meditation is to develop spiritual and emotional muscle, as though you are going to sit on top of a mountain and feel the power and strength of it underneath you. In truth, you are going to feel your own power and strength. You are going to become your own mountain.

Once you have used "Sitting the Mountain" several times, and feel that you have developed some spiritual and emotional endurance, you are ready to move on to the next meditation in this chapter. "Prison of the Mind" is about judgment. Despite its unpleasant title, it is one of my most-requested meditations. This meditation will help you examine all the judgments that have been made about you by other people, and how you have developed ways to defend against them. Sometimes our defenses are not always healthy. By analyzing them, we can choose new and better ways to deal with judgment. The next meditation, "Transforming Judgment," will allow you to examine and transform the judgments you have of other people.

After working through the effects of judgment on your life, you will be ready to move on to the next meditation, "Dealing with Loss." This meditation will allow you to explore and heal a loss that you have experienced in the past, or one that you are going through now. This loss may have been a tangible loss through the death of a loved one, or a heart loss through emotional abandonment by a parent or lover. For example, if you are a man or woman whose ability to love depended upon an emotionally withdrawn father, you may continue to try to get the love you need by becoming involved in relationships with people who are emotionally withdrawn. You may even work for employers who are this way. Over and over again you give your love and loyalty to someone who does not reciprocate, and you are left feeling empty, lost, and abandoned, without understanding why. By doing the meditation, you may be able to get in touch with this original loss and feel your grief and anger toward your father, thereby breaking the cycle. You may even be able to forgive him when you see that he was a human being without the ability to love. When you come across people who don't have this ability, you will recognize them and stay away from them, or not take it personally when they can't fill your needs.

I have always told my students that you can't put icing on a burned cake, meaning that you can't cover up dark feelings with sweetness and light. Many people think that forgiveness is about sweetness and light. It's not. It is a very challenging, deep, and healing process. To forgive someone means to let go of the toxic feelings that keep us attached to the past and to people in it, while at the same time remembering what happened so that we don't allow it to happen again. The meditation "Heart Opening" will help you forgive someone who has hurt you. You may discover that it is more powerful to open your heart in compassion and forgiveness, thereby keeping it filled with strength and energy, than to try to keep it closed.

Forgiveness is tough love. It demands honesty with ourselves and with others. When we have done or said something that injures someone else, we have to make a choice between guilt and remorse. To feel guilty is to choose the road that leads to constant self-reproach and a replaying, over and over again, of the injurious situation in our minds. In the end, it doesn't accomplish anything. There is no healing in guilt. The meditation entitled "Remorse," on the other hand, will help you experience a deep sadness in your heart for the choices you have made and the actions you have taken. It is like looking directly into a mirror of truth that can open to healing and self-forgiveness.

Self-forgiveness is sometimes the hardest to accomplish. We don't always believe that we have a right to our anger, our needs, or our actions that attempt to fill those needs—as though other people are more important, and we are less so. We blame ourselves for our weaknesses and imperfections, holding ourselves to a higher standard than other people. "Self-Forgiveness" will help you open your heart to yourself and heal the wounds of your own self-judgment and self-punishment. Over the years, my students have said many times that it is one of their favorite meditations.

Once you have practiced "Self-Forgiveness," and feel that most of your self-reproach is behind you, you may wish to use "Self-Love" on a daily basis. In forgiving ourselves and forgiving others, we can open our hearts to true healing. No longer will our minds be filled with the replaying of conflicts. No longer will our bodies have to suffer the confusion of mixed signals and toxic emotions. No longer will we have to keep our hearts closed. In cleansing and balancing our bodies and souls, minds and hearts, we can come to the most healing place of all: self-love.

Sitting the Mountain

✢ *This meditation will help you build spiritual and emotional endurance, as well as establish physical grounding. It is a good meditation to work with before attempting to try any of the other meditations in this chapter. Allow yourself to drop down deeply into your body and awareness. Do not attempt to change anything you are experiencing. Take your time. This is a fairly brief meditation, but it has powerful and healing results that build with continuous use.*

Find a comfortable position, either sitting or lying down. Uncross your arms and legs, and close your eyes. Take a long, deep breath, and let it out slowly. Allow your breathing to become full, deep, and relaxed.

As you count from ten to zero, allow your rational mind to rest, and you will become more receptive to the wisdom of your soul and its healing power: ten–nine–eight–seven–six–five–four–three–two–one–zero. You are now very deeply relaxed.

Allow yourself to settle into your body. Allow any extraneous noises to float past you.

Retain your awareness within. Breathe.

Settle into your body so that your body becomes your support, your mountain.

Feel your shoulders and neck relax. Your forehead and jaw soften. Allow all the muscles, nerves, and organs to become peaceful.

When you are comfortable in your body, allow yourself to become deeply still within.

Breathe deeply, and focus your attention on your breath.

Allow yourself to become aware of an issue in your life that causes you great pain.

Become fully aware of, and remain present with, this pain . . . physically, emotionally, mentally, and spiritually.

Surrender to it. Drop down into it. Be absolutely fearless in the face of this pain.

Allow yourself to observe, feel, hear, and know everything about this pain.

Allow yourself to become aware of the transformation and healing that your own consciousness brings to this issue.

Become aware of the strength and endurance that you are building as you face into the truth of what you are feeling.

Allowing yourself to remain in touch with your feelings, very slowly, whenever you feel ready, you may open your eyes after the count of ten: one–two–three–four–five–six–seven–eight–nine–ten.

Prison of the Mind

✤ *This meditation will allow you to examine the judgments that you have experienced from other people since your childhood. You will be able to notice how you defend against these judgments, and then choose different responses that will be more effective.*

Find a comfortable position, either sitting or lying down. Uncross your arms and legs, and close your eyes. Take a long, deep breath, and let it out slowly. Allow your breathing to become full, deep, and relaxed.

As you count from ten to zero, allow your rational mind to rest, and you will become more receptive to the wisdom of your soul and its healing power: ten–nine–eight–seven–six–five–four–three–two–one–zero. You are now very deeply relaxed.

Image yourself standing or sitting in the middle of a prison cell without doors or windows. There is enough fresh air to breathe easily.

Now look up at the ceiling. As you do, you begin to notice an image of the people who have been involved in your spiritual development. Behind them, written on the ceiling, are all the judgments that you have received from them.

Allow yourself to see them as clearly as possible, and read the judgments, one by one. As you do, notice how your body feels.

How have these judgments affected your life?

How have you attempted to defend yourself against their judgments?

Now take a long, deep breath. Allow yourself to let go of all the ways that you usually defend yourself. Release any tensions in your body and arguments in your mind. Breathe.

Allow yourself to see them as they really are: human beings with their own pain, their own self-judgments, who are separate from you. Feel this separateness. Feel your own, individual identity.

Now let go of this image of them. Take a deep breath, and begin to wipe off the ceiling with your mind. If you wish, imagine taking a white cloth and wiping off the ceiling by hand. As you do, notice it dissolving in front of your eyes.

When you are finished, the ceiling is gone and an open space remains. Feel this freedom. Breathe deeply.

Now face one of the walls. As you do, you begin to notice an image of your mother forming, and behind her, written on the wall, are all the judgments that you have received from her.

Allow yourself to see her as clearly as possible, and read the judgments, one by one. As you do, notice how your body feels.

How have these judgments affected your life?

How have you attempted to defend yourself against her judgments?

Now take a long, deep breath. Allow yourself to let go of all the ways that you usually defend yourself. Release any tension in your body and arguments in your mind. Breathe.

Allow yourself to see your mother as she really is: a human being with her own pain, her own self-judgments, someone who is separate from you. Feel this separateness. Feel your own, individual identity.

Now let go of this image of your mother. Take a deep breath and begin to wipe off the wall with your mind. If you wish, imagine taking a white cloth and wiping down the wall by hand. As you do, notice the wall dissolving in front of your eyes.

When you are finished, the wall is gone, and open space remains. Feel this freedom. Breathe deeply.

Now turn to the next wall on your right. As you face this wall, you begin to notice an image of your father forming, and behind him, written on the wall, are all the judgments that you have received from him.

Allow yourself to see him as clearly as possible, and read the judgments, one by one. As you do, notice how your body feels.

How have these judgments affected your life?

How have you attempted to defend yourself against his judgments?

Now take a long, deep breath. Allow yourself to let go of all the ways that you usually defend yourself. Release any tensions in your body and arguments in your mind. Breathe.

Allow yourself to see your father as he really is: a human being with his own pain, his own self-judgments, someone who is separate from you. Feel this separateness. Feel your own, individual identity.

Now let go of this image of your father. Take a deep breath and begin to wipe off the wall with your mind. If you wish, imagine taking a white cloth and wiping down the wall by hand. As you do, notice the wall dissolving in front of your eyes.

When you are finished, the wall is gone and an open space remains. Feel this freedom. Breathe deeply.

Now turn to the next wall on your right. As you face this wall, you begin to notice an image forming of other family members and friends, and behind them, written on the wall, are all the judgments that you have received from them.

Allow yourself to see them as clearly as possible, and read the judgments, one by one. As you do, notice how your body feels.

How have these judgments affected your life?

How have you attempted to defend yourself against their judgments?

Now take a long, deep breath. Allow yourself to let go of all the ways that you usually defend yourself. Release any tensions in your body and arguments in your mind. Breathe.

Allow yourself to see your family and friends as they really are: human beings with their own pain, their own self-judgments, people who are separate from you. Feel this separateness. Feel your own, individual identity.

Now let go of this image of your family and friends. Take a deep breath and begin to wipe off the wall with your mind. If you wish, imagine taking a white cloth and wiping down the wall by hand. As you do, notice the wall dissolving in front of your eyes.

When you are finished, the wall is gone and an open space remains. Feel this freedom. Breathe deeply.

Now turn to the next wall on your right. As you face this wall, you begin to notice an image forming of people you have known in your education and career, and behind them, written on the wall, are all the judgments that you have received from them.

Allow yourself to see them as clearly as possible, and read the judgments, one by one. As you do, notice how your body feels.

How have these judgments affected your life?

How have you attempted to defend yourself against their judgments?

Now take a long, deep breath. Allow yourself to let go of all the ways that you usually defend yourself. Release any tensions in your body and arguments in your mind. Breathe.

Allow yourself to see these people as they really are: as human beings with their own pain, their own self-judgments, people who are separate from you. Feel this separateness. Feel your own, individual identity.

Now let go of this image of them. Take a deep breath and begin to wipe off the wall with your mind. If you wish, imagine taking a white cloth and wiping down the wall by hand. As you do, notice the wall dissolving in front of your eyes.

When you are finished, the wall is gone and an open space remains. Feel this freedom. Breathe deeply.

Now turn to the floor under your feet. As you face downward, you begin to notice an image forming of yourself, and behind you, written on the floor, are all your self-judgments.

Allow yourself to see this image as clearly as possible, and read the judgments, one by one. As you do, notice how your body feels.

How have these judgments affected your life?

How have you attempted to defend yourself against your own judgments?

Now take a long, deep breath. Allow yourself to let go of all the ways that you usually defend yourself. Release any tensions in your body and arguments in your mind. Breathe.

Now see yourself as you really are: a human being who has absorbed many judgments from other people. Which of your own self-judgments have some truth to them—truth that is worth saving?

Which judgments are false and distorted?

Which judgments is it time to let go of?

Take a deep breath, and begin to wipe off the judgments that you desire to release. In their place, write down some constructive truths about yourself.

When you are finished, stand up and feel the solidity and security of this ground underneath your feet. Breathe.

Remaining aware of the truth and ground under your feet, you may open your eyes on the count of ten: one–two–three–four–five–six–seven–eight–nine–ten.

Transforming Judgment

✤ *This meditation will allow you to examine and transform the judgments you have about other people.*

Find a comfortable position, either sitting or lying down. Uncross your arms and legs, and close your eyes. Take a long, deep breath, and let it out slowly. Allow your breathing to become full, deep, and relaxed.

As you count from ten to zero, allow your rational mind to rest, and you will become more receptive to the wisdom of your unconscious and its healing power: ten–nine–eight–seven–six–five–four–three–two–one–zero. You are now very deeply relaxed.

Image your mother sitting or standing in front of you. See her as clearly as possible, and notice how you feel in her presence.

What judgments do you have about your mother?

Which of these judgments have anger?

Sadness?

Fear?

Now take a long, deep breath. Look deeply into your mother's eyes and see her clearly, as a human being with a history and childhood of her own. See her struggle, her pain, her weaknesses.

See her strength, her love, her life force.

Release your attachment to your own emotions of fear, sadness, and anger.

Seeing your mother more clearly, which of your judgments need to be transformed?

Which of your judgments have truth to them?

Now take a deep breath. Allow yourself to change your former judgments into statements of truth.

As you look once more at your mother, does she appear any different to you?

Now gently release your mother.

Image your father sitting or standing in front of you. See him as clearly as possible, and notice how you feel in his presence.

What judgments do you have about your father?

Which of these judgments have anger?

Sadness?

Fear?

Now take a long, deep breath. Look deeply into your father's eyes and see him clearly, as a human being with a history and childhood of his own. See his struggle, his pain, his weaknesses.

See his strength, his love, his life force.

Release your attachment to your own emotions of fear, sadness, and anger.

Seeing your father more clearly, which of your judgments need to be transformed?

Which of your judgments have truth to them?

Now take a deep breath. Allow yourself to change your former judgments into statements of truth.

As you look once more at your father, does he appear any different to you?

Now gently release your father.

Image other family members and friends sitting or standing in front of you. See them as clearly as possible, and notice how you feel in their presence.

What judgments do you have about your family and friends?

Which of these judgments have anger?

Sadness?

Fear?

Now take a long, deep breath. Look deeply into their eyes and see them clearly, as human beings with histories and childhoods of their own. See their struggles, their pain, their weaknesses.

See their strengths, their love, their life force.

Release your attachment to your own emotions of fear, sadness, and anger.

Seeing your family and friends more clearly, which of your judgments need to be transformed?

Which of your judgments have truth to them?

Take a deep breath. Allow yourself to change your former judgments into statements of truth.

As you look once more at these people, do they appear any different to you?

Now gently release them.

Image people from your education and career sitting or standing in front of you. See them as clearly as possible, and notice how you feel in their presence.

What judgments do you have about them?

Which of these judgments have anger?

Sadness?

Fear?

Now take a long, deep breath. Look deeply into their eyes and see them clearly, as human beings with histories and childhoods of their own. See their struggle, their pain, their weaknesses.

See their strength, their love, their life force.

Release your attachment to your own emotions of fear, sadness, and anger.

Now seeing them more clearly, which of your judgments need to be transformed?

Which of your judgments have truth to them?

Now take a deep breath. Allow yourself to change your former judgments into statements of truth.

As you look once more at these people, do they appear any different to you?

Now gently release them.

Image people involved in your religious upbringing and your present spiritual life sitting or standing in front of you. See them as clearly as possible, and notice how you feel in their presence.

What judgments do you have about them?

Which of these judgments have anger?

Sadness?

Fear?

Now take a long, deep breath. Look deeply into their eyes and see them clearly, as human beings with histories and childhoods of their own. See their struggles, their pain, their weaknesses.

See their strength, their love, their life force.

Release your attachment to your own emotions of fear, sadness, and anger.

Seeing these people more clearly, which of your judgments need to be transformed?

Which judgments have truth to them?

Now take a deep breath. Allow yourself to change your former judgments into statements of truth.

As you look once more at these people, do they appear any different to you?

Now gently release them.

And finally, image yourself sitting or standing in front of you. See yourself as clearly as possible, and notice how you feel.

What judgments do you have about yourself?

Which of these judgments have anger?

Sadness?

Fear?

Now take a long, deep breath. Look deeply into your own eyes and see yourself clearly, as a human being with a history and childhood of your own. See your struggles, your pain, your weaknesses.

See your strength, your love, your life force.

Release your attachment to your own emotions of fear, sadness, and anger.

Seeing yourself more clearly, which of your judgments need to be transformed?

Which judgments have truth to them?

Now take a deep breath. Allow yourself to change your former judgments into statements of truth.

As you look once more at yourself, do you appear any different?

Take a long, deep breath and notice how you feel. Allow yourself to experience the freedom and openness that comes with releasing judgment and embracing truth.

On the count of ten you may open your eyes: one–two–three–four–five–six–seven–eight–nine–ten.

Dealing with Loss

✤ *This meditation will assist you in healing the losses that you have experienced in your life. You may use it to help heal grief from the loss of someone through death or the ending of a relationship. You can resolve emotional abandonment in your childhood, or losses that you are experiencing currently. Some people even use this meditation to help heal the loss of a beloved pet. This is a deep meditation and is best used when you are alone and have time to remain with your feelings for a while after the meditation is complete. Before you begin, choose the person or pet that you wish to focus on during the meditation. If there are several, use the meditation separately for each one.*

Find a comfortable position, either sitting or lying down. Uncross your arms and legs, and close your eyes. Take a long, deep breath, and let it out slowly. Allow your breathing to become full, deep, and relaxed.

As you count from ten to zero, allow your rational mind to rest, and you will become more receptive to the wisdom of your soul and its healing power: ten–nine–eight–seven–six–five–four–three–two–one–zero. You are now very deeply relaxed.

Allow yourself to image someone you have lost. See them as clearly as possible, either sitting or standing in front of you.

Look into their eyes and feel their presence. Breathe.

Allow yourself to fully experience your sadness and grief at the loss of this loved one.

Stay in touch with your heart, your breathing, and how your body feels.

Notice where in your body you are feeling the most grief.

Now allow yourself to experience any guilt you feel in relationship to this person.

Stay in touch with your heart, your breathing, and your body.

Notice where in your body you are feeling the most guilt.

Now allow yourself to experience any anger you feel toward this person.

Stay in touch with your heart, your breathing, and your body.

Notice where in your body you are feeling the most anger.

Take a long, deep breath, and let it out slowly. As you do, begin to release the emotions of grief, guilt, and anger from your body.

Allow yourself to image a bright, white light, shimmering and shining out in the heavens, above your head. Imagine this light shining down all around you and through you.

As this light enters your body, allow it to help you heal and release the emotions of sadness, guilt, and anger. Allow this light to begin the cleansing process of releasing the past.

Imagine this white light flowing into the middle of your chest, where your heart center of love and compassion exists. Feel it filling your heart and flowing in a circular motion.

If you feel ready to forgive this person for any pain they have caused you, imagine this white light turning to a soft pink, the higher energy of the heart and the color of forgiveness.

Feel and see this pink light extending out to the other person and gently flowing into their heart. Breathe.

See this person receiving the light, love, forgiveness, and healing you are sending them.

Allow yourself to feel the connection of compassion and forgiveness that you have in this moment.

Allow this connection to melt any sense of loss you had, and feel the healing energy flowing back full circle into your heart again.

There is now a circle of pink light flowing through and between the two of you, connecting you on a deep spiritual level.

Knowing the strength of your connection, allow yourself to bid farewell to this person. Breathe. Image the light gently separating at a place between the two of you, with equal amounts moving back into your hearts.

Knowing that you are full with this light and love, gently release their image.

Retaining your awareness of this deep healing, you may open your eyes on the count of ten: one–two–three–four–five–six–seven–eight–nine–ten.

Heart Opening

❧ *This meditation will assist you in opening your heart to someone you feel the need to forgive. Remember that forgiveness is not about condoning what someone has done. To forgive someone means to see them clearly, truthfully, and then to let go of the past so that it does not control your future.*

Find a comfortable position, either sitting or lying down. Uncross your arms and legs, and close your eyes. Take a long, deep breath, and let it out slowly. Allow your breathing to become full, deep, and relaxed.

As you count from ten to zero, allow your rational mind to rest, and you will become more receptive to the wisdom of your soul and its healing power: ten–nine–eight–seven six–five–four–three–two–one–zero. You are now very deeply relaxed.

Allow yourself to image someone who often causes you to close your heart. See this person as clearly as possible, either sitting or standing in front of you.

Notice how you feel in this person's presence.

How does your body feel?

Notice your breathing. What emotions are you feeling?

What is it about this person that causes you to close your heart?

Is there anything you are afraid of?

Is there any way that you try to defend yourself?

What causes you to close your heart in this person's presence?

Now take a long, deep breath, and see if you can begin to release whatever you are afraid of, whatever you are angry about.

Allow yourself to release from your body and heart all the negative energies and emotions that you have previously been feeling toward this person.

Focus your attention way above the top of your head, out into the heavens, and get in touch with a very brilliant, sparkling, white light, like a star.

Feel this light energy coming down in a gentle stream all around you and through you.

Open yourself to receive this light energy, and feel it beginning to flow around you and through your body. Breathe it into your lungs, and feel it entering your heart.

Allow your heart, your center of love and compassion, to begin to open with this light energy, and feel it flowing in a circular motion in the middle of your chest.

As you continue to breathe deeply, feel your heart growing stronger with compassion.

Gradually open your heart wider and wider, feeling the strength of its energy beginning to permeate your entire body.

Feel it flowing down through your torso into your legs and feet.

Up through your shoulders, arms, and hands.

Feel your spine filling with light energy.

Now allow yourself to have the courage to clearly see this person in front of you. See this person's humanity: the weaknesses, failures, fears, anger, sadness, loss.

See the decisions that he or she has made, and the ways that they have hurt you.

See this person as he or she must have been as a newborn baby, still innocent and beautiful.

Allow yourself to keep your heart open. Breathe deeply, and feel the strength and compassion in your heart.

Allow your heart to fill with compassion, forgiveness, and healing.

Continue to experience a growing forgiveness and compassion until your heart expands further than you ever believed possible.

Feel your entire being filled with the light of forgiveness.

Experience yourself radiating light and compassion, healing and forgiveness. Open-hearted and powerful, feel yourself letting go of the past.

Feel your whole being so filled with the power of forgiveness that it flows out from you to the other person and heals the relationship.

You can create healing by your presence, a presence filled with forgiveness.

Knowing that the healing power of forgiveness will continue in your heart, you may release the other person's image.

You may open your eyes on the count of ten: one–two–three–four–five–six–seven–eight–nine–ten.

Remorse

✤ *This meditation will help you transform guilt into the healing power of remorse. It is a strong self-healing meditation that can erase past mistakes, and allow you to take actions that will permanently heal your self-image and your relationships with other people.*

Find a comfortable position, either sitting or lying down. Uncross your arms and legs, and close your eyes. Take a long, deep breath, and let it out slowly. Allow your breathing to become full, deep, and relaxed.

As you count down from ten to zero, allow your rational mind to rest, and you will become more receptive to the wisdom of your soul and its healing power: ten—nine—eight—seven—six—five—four—three—two—one—zero. You are now very deeply relaxed.

Image yourself standing in front of a very fancy, gilded, full-length mirror. Look carefully at its intricate frame.

Now look into the mirror and see the image that you present to the world. Examine all the intricacies of this image.

What qualities and characteristics seem to be coming through this image in the mirror? Is this how you want people to see you?

How do you keep up this image? What defenses do you use?

How do you hide your feelings when you have said or done something that you feel bad about?

Now take a deep breath and let go. Imagine closing your eyes to this mirror. Take a large step to your left. When you open your eyes again, you will be standing in front of a different mirror, the mirror of your true self. Open your eyes. What do you see now?

Look directly into this mirror. Face into its truth. What do you see?

What qualities and characteristics do you keep hidden from the outside world?

Look carefully at the frame of this mirror. How is it different from the other frame?

Now look into the center of the mirror at yourself. Are there any actions you have taken, or words you have said, that you feel guilty about?

Now take a deep breath. As you do, allow yourself to drop down into your heart in the middle of your chest. Drop down into your center of love and compassion, and allow yourself to feel the sadness underneath the guilt. Breathe.

Allow yourself to feel the deep remorse that accompanies being human. Allow yourself to feel your vulnerability, imperfections, and mistakes.

Allow yourself to admit, in your own heart, the ways that you have betrayed yourself and others.

And now, become aware of how you would like to heal these relationships.

What actions could you take? What words could you speak?

What would it take for you to begin to heal the past and the present?

Now image yourself doing whatever is necessary to heal the relationship with yourself and your relationships with others.

Imagine yourself asking forgiveness from each person you have injured. (Pause for sixty seconds.)

Now look directly into the mirror, and ask yourself for forgiveness. What is your response?

Now take a long, deep breath, and feel the healing that is beginning in your heart. The healing power of truth, remorse, and forgiveness.

Sit as long as you wish and, only when you feel ready, you may open your eyes after the count of ten: one–two–three–four–five–six–seven–eight–nine–ten.

Self-Forgiveness

✦ *This meditation will assist you in releasing the past, letting go of guilt and shame, and healing your heart. Self-forgiveness is an essential part of the healing process, as it opens the heart with love and healing energy. During this meditation you will have the opportunity to experience this energy in your own hands, and to do a brief laying-on-of-hands with your heart.*

Find a comfortable position, either sitting or lying down. Uncross your arms and legs, and close your eyes. Take a long, deep breath, and let it out slowly. Allow your breathing to become full, deep, and relaxed.

As you count down from ten to zero, allow your rational mind to rest, and you will become more receptive to the wisdom of your soul and its healing power: ten–nine–eight–seven–six–five–four–three–two–one–zero. You are now very deeply relaxed.

Focus your attention far above the top of your head, out into the heavens, and get in touch with a brilliant, powerful, white light and energy flowing down toward you.

Allow yourself to experience this light energy flowing all around you and through you, filling your body with its radiance.

With each breath, you inhale this light. As it fills and surrounds you, it gently permeates your entire being and joins the river of life energy already flowing through your body.

Allow your attention to focus this white light in the middle of your chest, in your center of love and compassion, your heart chakra. Feel it gently moving in a circular motion and opening your heart.

Breathe. Allow your heart to fill and open with love and compassion, light and radiance.

Now visualize yourself seated in front of you. See yourself as clearly as possible, as though looking in a mirror or at a photograph.

Allow yourself to see and feel all your flaws, fears, anger, guilt, and shame: all the things that keep you from self-love.

See all the ways you try to protect and defend yourself.

See all the ways in which you fail to live up to your own expectations.

Send the white light of compassion and self-love out from your heart across to you, and see it entering your heart and being received.

Feel and see this love light flowing through you and out to this other you, entering your heart and being received.

Allow yourself to forgive yourself.

Allow this self-forgiveness to heal the wounds of your heart with new light and self-love.

Now switch roles and become the other you, the one who is being forgiven.

Feel this forgiveness and light entering your heart.

Feel the gentle healing power of this forgiveness and love, and allow yourself to feel blessed.

Allow this white light and love to pour through you, pour through your whole body: all the way down into your torso, legs, and feet.

Up into your throat and neck, face and head.

Down through your shoulders, arms, and hands.

Allow this love light to pour through you, cleansing you, healing you, releasing you.

And now, keeping your eyes closed, focus this light in your hands.

Very gently lift your hands and bring them up until they are about 10 or 12 inches apart, palms facing each other. Relax your hands and fingers.

Move your hands toward each other until you can feel the energy between your two palms.

This is the energy of healing, love, and forgiveness. This energy is tangible and real. It is your participation in Creation.

Keeping your eyes closed, bring your hands up to your head, so that your palms are several inches from your face.

Move your hands toward your face until you can feel the energy between your hands and face.

And then, very slowly, bring them down in front of your throat.

And over your chest where your heart rests.

Feel the contact of energy between your hands and your heart. Breathe.

As you now forgive yourself, you participate in the atonement and peace of your own heart.

And the atonement and peace of all Creation.

Allow yourself to stay in this deep state of healing as long as you wish. After the count of ten, you may open your eyes when you are ready: one–two–three–four–five–six–seven–eight–nine–ten.

Self-Love

✤ *This meditation will assist you in getting in touch with the eternal light of Creation alive within your heart, the healing power of self-love. It is a wonderful meditation to do on a daily basis.*

Find a comfortable position, either sitting or lying down. Uncross your arms and legs, and close your eyes. Take a long, deep breath, and let it out slowly. Allow your breathing to become full, deep, and relaxed.

As you count down from ten to zero, allow your rational mind to rest, and you will become more receptive to the wisdom of your soul and its healing power: ten–nine–eight–seven–six–five–four–three–two–one–zero. You are now very deeply relaxed.

Drop down, deeply within. Drop down into your heart, and breathe.

Drop down into the quiet, still place within you. Down inside the very center of your heart, the very center of love and compassion.

Take your hands and place them over your heart. As you breathe deeply, allow your heart to open from the inside.

As your heart opens, you can feel and see the eternal light of Creation beginning to shine forth through the darkness.

All the dark, rejected, abandoned parts of you begin to move aside as this light grows larger and brighter.

This inner Divinity, the eternal flame of love, is at the very center of your being. Feel this flame grow brighter and brighter as your heart opens.

Allow yourself to feel the warmth of this flame flowing out from your heart and through your entire body, filling you with light and love.

As this love flows through every cell of your body, feel its healing presence.

Feel it flowing out from your heart and into your arms and hands, and then back into your heart.

Feel this deep love, self-love, as you give and receive the light of Creation. All this love, healing, and light, contained within you, flowing out from you and back into you.

Become aware of the healing of this self-love, your acceptance of who you are, the light and the dark making peace with each other.

Allow this self-love to so permeate your soul, your body, your entire being, that you create a deep peace within you.

Remain as long as you wish in the center of self-love. After the count of ten, you may open your eyes when you are ready: one–two–three–four–five–six–seven–eight–nine–ten.

CHAPTER 3
Psychic Self-Defense

Finding Your Weak Link

Sourcing Your Self-Image

Unhooking

Psychic Self-Defense Affirmations

Seeing with a Dark Eye

Strengthening Your Aura

Boundaries

$\mathcal{W}$e spend most of our day in other people's energy fields. Many of us sleep next to someone else, eat our meals in the presence of our families, friends, and coworkers, and sit next to colleagues at our jobs. If we live in a big city, just walking down the street means that we are surrounded by hundreds of strangers every day.

When we get home from work, not only do we encounter our families and friends, but we often turn on the television or radio, and read the newspaper. If we work at home, we may be bombarded by the energy of our children, or the television, all day long. Most people spend very little, if any, time in solitude. In fact, many people consider solitude to be "lonely," and try to avoid being alone at all costs. They don't realize how high the cost really is.

Being around other people all day and night means that we hardly ever have a chance to renew our own individual energy field. Each one of us is a special being with its own life force. We have a completely unique body, emotional makeup, set of thoughts, and spiritual development. We have more than one body of energy (see chapter 1, "Healing Your Body"). Even our chakras, the subtle energy centers in our etheric body, are in states of strength or weakness that are particular to each of us.

When we do nothing to safeguard and maintain the integrity of our individual energy field, we leave ourselves vulnerable to absorbing and being affected by the energies of others and our environment. This can have deleterious effects on our physical health, as well as our emotional, mental, and spiritual well-being. When I was a child, I was very sensitive to other people's emotions and thoughts. I could tell what someone was feeling just by looking at them, and I would often experience their emotions and even their physical condition in my own body. I was what I call a *psychic sponge*. I would soak up the other person's energies and experience them as my own. Constantly surrounded by family members who were physically ill, I likewise found myself getting sick. I never developed firm boundaries of protection.

If you are a psychic sponge, you may notice similar reactions. You may find that you are aware of how someone is feeling as soon as you see them. You may think it is just because you can read it on the person's face, but not everyone has a face that gives away inner feelings. It is probably more than this. You are most likely feeling, *clairsentiently,* the energy coming off the person's body and aura, or energy field. *Clairsentience* means "clear feeling." In Great Britain, psychics are called *sensitives.* If you are sensitive in this physical and emotional way, then you are more vulnerable than most people to absorbing and experiencing other people's illnesses, emotions, and thoughts. For example, if you have lunch with a friend who is going through a divorce, much of the time may be spent talking about the divorce proceedings and your friend's negative feelings. At the end of the lunch, your friend may feel much relieved, while you go home or back to work with an upset stomach and feeling "down." You felt fine before lunch, but you "ate" your friend's angry words and sat for an hour in this toxic energy. Maybe it even stirred up negative feelings from your own divorce several years ago, or similar feelings you are having toward someone you know.

Another example is that most people don't like to go to hospitals to visit the sick, and may feel guilty because they consider their reaction irrational. After all, we aren't actually going to catch anything, are we? But these fears are not completely unfounded. There are dozens, sometimes hundreds, of people who are sick and dying within any one hospital. Many people are in physical pain, as well as emotional, mental, and spiritual distress. If you are especially sensitive, you may indeed feel more than you want to feel when you walk into a hospital. People working in hospitals, like nurses, doctors, and technicians, are exposed to these negative energies every day, as well as to the electromagnetic fields (EMFs) that are emitted by all the technology. These fields operate at a different resonant frequency than the human body, and can affect it over a period of time. You may find yourself feeling more tired than usual, or the reverse, unable to sleep. If you are sensitive to energy, you may find that you feel the effects of these electromagnetic fields whether you notice them or not.

How do we protect ourselves from all these energetic assaults? By finding ways to maintain and safeguard the integrity of our personal energy field. The most important way to start is to find some time to be in solitude, at least three times a day, more often if you need to. Early in the morning, after getting up, is a good time, because you can assess how you feel before the day begins to get too hectic. Sit quietly, breathe, and allow yourself to become aware of how you feel. Ask yourself these questions: How does my body feel right now? How do I feel emotionally? What thoughts and concerns are on my mind? Are these affecting my body in any way? Later in the day, maybe late morning, lunch time, or in the middle of the afternoon, sit quietly for a few minutes and do the same thing. It takes only a few minutes, but you will begin to get a sense of how the activities of the day, and the people in it, have affected you. Then again at night, either when you get home from work, or before going to bed, sit and notice how you feel. Ask yourself: How do I feel now? How does this compare with how I felt when I woke up? As you do this, you will begin to notice more subtle differences between morning, afternoon, and evening. You will begin to be able to distinguish what events and which people have most affected your individual energy system. This is called *recognizing,* and is the first step of Psychic Self-Defense.

There are two meditations here that will help you recognize why you are so vulnerable to people and the environment: "Finding Your Weak Link" and "Sourcing Your Self-Image." The first will have you image a situation in which you feel negatively affected by some-one, help you notice how they are injuring you, and then guide you to insights about other people and occurrences that are similar. The second meditation will help you trace back in your childhood to the people who imprinted you with negative self-images, and assist you in *releasing* those images.

Releasing is step two of Psychic Self-Defense: letting go of other people's negative energies, the energies of your environment, and even those feelings inside you that may be weakening your well-being. When you return from having lunch with that friend who is getting divorced, you could sit for three minutes, recognize how you feel different from the way you did before lunch, and then release all the sadness (and indigestion). "Unhooking" is a good meditation for this situation, as it takes you through all seven chakras, noticing where you have gotten hooked by someone else's energy, emotions, or thoughts. If you don't have time to do all seven chakras before you go back to work, you could choose just one, your stomach!

Once you have released whatever you don't want, you can then move on to step three, *repairing.* That sense of depletion you may be feeling after lunch is not only because of your friend's anger and your indigestion, but because the situation has literally stolen your life force. The positive feelings and healthy energy you had before lunch have been depleted in the course of being assaulted by your friend's negative feelings and your participation in the discussion and situation. Maybe you sympathized with him or her. Maybe you began to resonate with this person. In physics, *to resonate with* means to vibrate at the same frequency, just like an atom or electron. No wonder you feel awful. Repairing the damage entails finding your own energy frequency once again and keeping it intact. The meditations "Strengthening Your Aura" and "Psychic Self-Defense Affirmations" can help you do this.

These last two meditations are also valuable in *protection and prevention,* step four of Psychic Self-Defense. Once you have *recognized* why you are so vulnerable to the energies around you, *released* whatever is not yours, and *repaired* the damage to your energy field, you need to *protect* yourself and *prevent* further occurrences from debilitating you. This means "Seeing with a Dark Eye" and developing strong "Boundaries." When we see someone with a dark eye, it means that we are willing to see the shadow hiding beneath the person's personality. It means that we are willing to look underneath whatever persona the person is trying to present to the world: the smiling face, the pleasantries, the "good" person. It is not that the persona is completely false. It is just that these positive qualities are not the whole person. Everyone has a dark side of unresolved sadness, fear, anger, and guilt. When we are willing to see this unhealed portion of someone, we stand a better chance of being able to protect ourselves when it finally reveals itself. If we are not willing to see this shadow, then it can catch us off guard when we least expect it.

If someone catches us off guard, we may feel that the person has invaded our boundaries. We can stay conscious of maintaining a strong sense of self by using either the "Strengthening Your Aura" meditation or the "Boundaries" meditation every morning before we leave our home. Most of us feel more protected in our own home than we do in the world. By doing one of these two meditations every morning, exercising, and eating in a healthy way, we develop strength in physical and psychic ways that can be better maintained during the day. In the evening, doing the "Unhooking" meditation can release the energies that we may have absorbed or collected.

Psychic Self-Defense is a lifelong spiritual practice. The stronger, more protected, and healthier you become, the more you will find that life can be lived with clarity and intention, love and forgiveness, grounding and security. It is up to you to put these exercises into effect. Imagine yourself as a spiritual warrior, with the right and the courage to protect the life that God has given you.

Finding Your Weak Link

✤ *This meditation will assist you in discovering why you are vulnerable to other people's negative energies. You will have the opportunity to explore present relationships, as well as make connections to the past. By the end of the meditation, you may find that you can begin to protect yourself and remain strong and centered.*

Find a comfortable position, either sitting or lying down. Uncross your arms and legs, and close your eyes. Take a long, deep breath, and let it out slowly. Allow your breathing to become full, deep, and relaxed.

As you count from ten to zero, allow your rational mind to rest, and you will become more receptive to the wisdom of your soul and its healing power: ten–nine–eight–seven–six five–four–three–two–one–zero. You are now very deeply relaxed.

Allow yourself to image a situation in which you felt vulnerable in the face of someone else's negative energy.

See this situation as clearly as possible and feel how you felt then.

What are you feeling emotionally?

Physically?

Where in your body are you responding to this person and situation?

How is it affecting you?

Is this situation similar to other situations that you have felt yourself in before? Does it remind you of anything or anyone in your childhood?

Who is this person to you?

What is your emotional connection with this person?

Is there something you need or want from this person?

Is there something you are afraid of?

What kind of energy does this person seem to be giving off or directing toward you?

What is the weak link in you that allows yourself to become hooked into this person's negative energy?

What do you need to let go of or resolve in yourself to remain unhooked?

Now visualize yourself resolving this inner conflict, and letting go of anything you need to release. Breathe.

Let go from all the places in your body where you have been holding tension or tightness.

As you take a long, deep breath, re-image the same situation, this time remaining centered and strong in the face of this other person.

Feel the difference in your emotions and your body as you confront the situation from a clear and neutral place.

Visualize yourself handling this situation and responding to this person in a healthy way.

Knowing that you can remain centered and strong in the future, you may release the image and open your eyes on the count of ten: one–two–three–four–five–six–seven–eight–nine–ten.

Sourcing Your Self-Image

❖ *This meditation will assist you in tracing the development of some of your self-images and the people involved in creating them. You will have the opportunity to release those self-images that you do not wish to keep.*

Find a comfortable position, either sitting or lying down. Uncross your arms and legs, and close your eyes. Take a long, deep breath, and let it out slowly. Allow your breathing to become full, deep, and relaxed.

As you count from ten to zero, allow your rational mind to rest, and you will become more receptive to the wisdom of your soul and its healing power: ten—nine—eight—seven—six—five—four—three—two—one—zero. You are now very deeply relaxed.

Allow your unconscious to give you an image of a time or situation in your life when you felt vulnerable and powerless.

See this image as clearly as possible, and feel how you felt then.

How does your body respond to this self-image?

On the count of three, you will see the face or get the name of the person who has contributed most to your developing this self-image: one—two—three.

Tell this person how you feel about this negative self-image and their participation in creating it.

Tell them anything you have always wanted to tell them. Breathe.

If you wish to release this self-image, then imagine it dissolving. Tell the other person that if they wish to keep this image of you, they may, but you have released it.

Once you have done this, clear your mind.

Now allow your unconscious to give you an image of a time or situation in your life when you felt rejected.

See this image as clearly as possible, and feel how you felt then.

How does your body respond to this self-image?

On the count of three, you will see the face or get the name of the person who has contributed most to your developing this self-image: one–two–three.

Tell this person how you feel about this negative self-image and their participation in creating it.

Tell them anything you have always wanted to tell them. Breathe.

If you wish to release this self-image, then imagine it dissolving. Tell the other person that if they wish to keep this image of you, they may, but you have released it.

Once you have done this, clear your mind.

Now allow your unconscious to give you an image of a time or situation in your life when you felt overwhelmed by someone else's energy.

See this image as clearly as possible, and feel how you felt then.

How does your body respond to this self-image?

On the count of three, you will see the face or get the name of the person who has contributed most to your developing this self-image: one–two–three.

Tell this person how you feel about this negative self-image and their participation in creating it.

Tell them anything you have always wanted to tell them. Breathe.

If you wish to release this self-image, then imagine it dissolving. Tell the other person that if they wish to keep this image of you, they may, but you have released it.

Once you have done this, clear your mind.

Now allow yourself to review all the images you have seen: images of yourself as vulnerable and powerless, rejected, and overwhelmed.

Are any of these images the same or similar?

Are any of the people the same?

Take a long, deep breath, and once again allow yourself to dissolve these images and release them.

In your mind's eye, begin to see an image of yourself as strong, courageous, and self-loving.

See this self-image surrounded by white-gold light.

Now place your consciousness inside this golden image and feel this new strength, courage, and self-love inside you.

Breathe this white-gold light into you, until it permeates your entire being.

Notice how your body feels with this new energy.

Staying in touch with this self-image and the feelings that accompany it, you may open your eyes on the count of ten: one–two–three–four–five–six–seven–eight–nine–ten.

Unhooking

✤ *This meditation will assist you in releasing people who are affecting, manipulating, or controlling your energy. By examining each chakra and its energy, you have the opportunity to clear it of outside influences and regain your own energy. It is an excellent meditation to do at the end of the day.*

Find a comfortable position, either sitting or lying down. Uncross your arms and legs, and close your eyes. Take a long, deep breath, and let it out slowly. Allow your breathing to become full, deep, and relaxed.

As you count from ten to zero, allow your rational mind to rest, and you will become more receptive to the wisdom of your soul and its healing power: ten–nine–eight–seven–six–five–four–three–two–one–zero. You are now very deeply relaxed.

Focus your attention far above the top of your head, out into the heavens, and get in touch with a brilliant, powerful, white light and energy flowing down toward you.

Allow yourself to experience this light energy flowing all around you and through you, filling your body with its radiance. With each breath, you inhale this light. As it fills and surrounds you, it gently permeates your entire being and joins the river of life energy already filling your body.

Focus your attention at the base of your spine, where your coccyx bone is located. This is your root chakra, your center of security, safety, and grounding in the physical world. Get in touch with the white light in your first chakra as it gently moves in a circular motion.

Feel this white light as energy flowing down through your legs and feet and into the ground, connecting you with Mother Earth.

Notice any sensations and emotions that arise as you connect with the physical nature of your body and Mother Earth.

On the count of three, you will spontaneously see the face or hear the name of a person who is hooked into this chakra—someone who is affecting, controlling, or manipulating your energy: one–two–three.

Imagine this person's energy as a hook that you take out with your astral hands, and give it back.

Tell this person that you wish to be free of their influence, and anything else that you need to tell them.

Now clear your mind except for the white light gently cleansing and filling this chakra.

Now gradually allow the energy in your first chakra to continue flowing upward in a spiral motion into your second chakra, in the center of your pelvis.

This is your center of sexuality and creative life force. As the light energy opens your second chakra, it moves gently in a circular motion.

Notice any sensations and emotions that arise as you connect with your sexuality and creative life force.

On the count of three, you will spontaneously see the face or hear the name of a person who is hooked into this chakra—someone who is affecting, controlling, or manipulating your energy: one–two–three.

Imagine this person's energy as a hook that you take out with your astral hands, and give it back.

Tell this person that you wish to be free of their influence, and anything else that you need to tell them.

Now clear your mind except for the white light gently cleansing and filling this chakra.

Now gradually allow the energy in your second chakra to continue flowing upward in a spiral motion into your third chakra, at your solar plexus between your rib cage.

This is your center of physical willpower, motivation, and vitality. As the light energy opens your third chakra, it moves gently in a circular motion.

Notice any sensations and emotions that arise as you connect with your physical willpower, motivation, and vitality.

On the count of three, you will spontaneously see the face or hear the name of a person who is hooked into this chakra—someone who is affecting, controlling, or manipulating your energy: one–two–three.

Imagine this person's energy as a hook that you take out with your astral hands, and give it back.

Tell this person that you wish to be free of their influence, and anything else that you need to tell them.

Now clear your mind except for the white light gently cleansing and filling this chakra.

Now gradually allow the energy in your third chakra to continue flowing upward in a spiral motion into your fourth chakra, your heart center in the middle of your chest.

This is your center of love and compassion. As the light energy opens your fourth chakra, it moves gently in a circular motion.

Notice any sensations and emotions that arise as you connect with your heart.

On the count of three, you will spontaneously see the face or hear the name of a person who is hooked into this chakra—someone who is affecting, controlling, or manipulating your energy: one—two—three.

Imagine this person's energy as a hook that you take out with your astral hands, and give it back.

Tell this person that you wish to be free of their influence, and anything else that you need to tell them.

Now clear your mind except for the white light gently cleansing and filling this chakra.

Now gradually allow the energy in your heart chakra to continue flowing upward in a spiral motion into your fifth chakra, in the center of your throat.

This is your center of self-expression. As the light energy opens your fifth chakra, it moves gently in a circular motion.

Notice any sensations and emotions that arise as you connect with your self-expression.

On the count of three, you will spontaneously see the face or hear the name of a person who is hooked into this chakra—someone who is affecting, controlling, or manipulating your energy: one—two—three.

Imagine this person's energy as a hook that you take out with your astral hands, and give it back.

Tell this person that you wish to be free of their influence, and anything else that you need to tell them.

Now clear your mind except for the white light gently cleansing and filling this chakra.

Now gradually allow the energy in your fifth chakra to continue flowing upward in a spiral motion into your sixth chakra, between your eyebrows.

This is your center of psychic sight and true vision. As the light energy opens your third eye, it moves gently in a circular motion.

Notice any sensations and emotions that arise as you connect with your ability to see clearly.

On the count of three, you will spontaneously see the face or hear the name of a person who is hooked into this chakra—someone who is affecting, controlling, or manipulating your energy: one–two–three.

Imagine this person's energy as a hook that you take out with your astral hands, and give it back.

Tell this person that you wish to be free of their influence, and anything else that you need to tell them.

Now clear your mind except for the white light gently cleansing and filling this chakra.

Now gradually allow the energy in your third eye to continue flowing upward in a spiral motion into your seventh chakra, at the crown of your head.

This is your center of spiritual consciousness and direct knowing. As the light energy opens your seventh chakra, it moves gently in a circular motion.

Notice any sensations and emotions that arise as you connect with your spiritual consciousness.

On the count of three, you will spontaneously see the face or hear the name of a person who is hooked into this chakra—someone who is affecting, controlling, or manipulating your energy: one–two–three.

Imagine this person's energy as a hook that you take out with your astral hands, and give it back.

Tell this person that you wish to be free of their influence, and anything else that you need to tell them.

Now clear your mind except for the white light gently cleansing and filling this chakra.

Now allow your awareness to slowly scan down through all of your chakras. Allow yourself to feel the energy slowly moving in a circular motion in each center.

Feel the openness, clarity, and new strength flowing through you, as you have reclaimed your energies.

When you reach your first chakra at the base of your spine, re-connect with the light energy moving down through your legs and feet to give you a feeling of grounding.

On the count of ten, you may open your eyes: one–two–three–four–five–six–seven–eight–nine–ten. Give yourself a minute or two to become accustomed to being back in the room with your eyes open.

Psychic Self-Defense Affirmations

�֎ *This meditation will assist you in changing old negative beliefs and feelings about yourself into new and positive ones. When linear affirmations are combined with guided images, both sides of the brain are engaged, and more energy is enlisted for healing. This meditation can be used for repairing your energies, as well as for protection and prevention.*

Find a comfortable position, either sitting or lying down. Uncross your arms and legs, and close your eyes. Take a long, deep breath, and let it out slowly. Allow your breathing to become full, deep, and relaxed.

As you count from ten to zero, allow your rational mind to rest, and you will become more receptive to the wisdom of your soul and its healing power: ten–nine–eight–seven–six–five–four–three–two–one–zero. You are now very deeply relaxed.

Allow your unconscious to give you an image of a time or situation in your life when you felt that you did not have the right to exist.

See this image as clearly as possible and feel how you felt then.

In a moment, you will have the opportunity to take in new healing affirmations. You may repeat them silently to yourself, or if alone, you may repeat them out loud. As you do, feel and see the image of yourself in this situation as transforming, along with the affirmations.

I have the right to exist in this universe.

My existence is an important part of the divine plan.

I have a divine mission to fulfill, and specific lessons to learn.

I can choose to survive all obstacles and hardships.

I and I alone can choose the quality of my life.

Breathe. Allow yourself to feel the truth and power of these affirmations within you.

Now clear your mind so you can move on to the next image.

Allow your unconscious to give you an image of a time or situation in your life when you felt that your identity was dependent upon someone else's approval.

See this image as clearly as possible and feel how you felt then.

Now take a long, deep breath and allow this old belief and your feelings to transform with the following affirmations: I choose to let go of the need for other people's approval.

I accept myself, including my strengths and weaknesses, mistakes and successes.

I have the right to act as my own mirror of love and approval.

I approve of myself and all that I am.

I have the right to ask my own questions and live my own answers.

I choose to love and respect my existence, as I would that of a valued friend.

My life is a gift from the Universe, and my life gives light to the Universe.

Breathe. Allow yourself to feel the truth and power of these affirmations within you.

Now clear your mind so you can move on to the next image.

Allow your unconscious to give you an image of a time or situation in your life when you felt that being powerful was impossible for you, or that to be powerful would be dangerous.

See this image as clearly as possible and feel how you felt then.

Now allow this old belief about yourself and your feelings to transform with the following affirmations: I have the right to be assertive in the expression of what I want.

It *is* possible for me to be both powerful and loved by others.

I choose to be powerful in positive, creative, and constructive ways.

I accept my innate power as a manifestation of the life force within me.

I have all the strength, integrity, and courage I will ever need.

I choose to protect my unique energies, and to safeguard my boundaries with the world.

Breathe. Allow yourself to feel the truth and power of these affirmations within you.

Retaining these new, positive beliefs and images, you may open your eyes on the count of ten: one–two–three–four–five–six–seven–eight–nine–ten.

Seeing with a Dark Eye

✤ *This meditation will train you in seeing both the light and dark sides of other people. In seeing the dark side, or shadow, of another person, you see what has been hidden. Opening and using your sixth chakra, known as the third eye, allows you to see clearly the truth of people and situations. In having this whole vision, you may find that you can protect yourself more easily in situations where you have felt previously vulnerable, and even prevent future instances from occurring.*

Find a comfortable position, either sitting or lying down. Uncross your arms and legs, and close your eyes. Take a long, deep breath, and let it out slowly. Allow your breathing to become full, deep, and relaxed.

As you count from ten to zero, allow your rational mind to rest, and you will become more receptive to the wisdom of your soul and its healing power: ten–nine–eight–seven–six–five–four–three–two–one–zero. You are now very deeply relaxed.

Focus your attention far above the top of your head, out into the heavens, and get in touch with a brilliant, powerful, white light and energy flowing down toward you.

Allow yourself to experience this light energy flowing all around you and through you, filling your body with its radiance. With each breath you inhale this light. As it fills and surrounds you, it gently permeates your entire being and joins the river of life energy already filling your body.

Now focus your attention on your third eye, your center of clear vision, between your eyebrows. Take a long, deep breath, and feel this white light energy flowing easily and gently in and out of your third eye.

As your third eye opens, image and feel this white light energy flowing in a circular motion between your eyebrows. As it does, it changes to a rich indigo, or bluish-purple, light.

Now allow yourself to image someone you live with, or someone you know well. Image this person as either sitting or standing in front of you.

Imagine yourself holding a clear quartz crystal in your hands, with the point of the crystal directed toward this person. Crystals refract, or break up, light energy into different lengths. As you point this crystal, you notice that the other person is separating into two people: one light and the other dark.

Look closely at these two people. What do you see?

Allow yourself to focus on the light side. What characteristics, emotions, and personality traits do you see in this light person?

Now focus on the dark side, the shadow. What hidden traits, emotions, and characteristics do you see?

Have you previously noticed this shadow? When? Where?

What did you do with your awareness of this person's shadow when you first noticed it?

Did it frighten you? Make you angry? Sad? Did you try to ignore it?

Now that you have seen this person's shadow, how can your relationship grow, change, and become healthier for both of you?

How can you protect yourself from this person's shadow?

Take a long, deep breath, and as you release it, point the crystal down into the ground and allow the person's two sides to come together again.

Once this person is whole, release this image.

Now image a person who is an acquaintance of yours—someone from work, school, or someone you have met recently. Image this person either sitting or standing in front of you.

Imagine yourself holding a clear quartz crystal in your hands, with the point of the crystal directed toward this person. As you point this crystal, you notice that the other person is separating into two people: one light and the other dark.

Look closely at these two people. What do you see?

Allow yourself to focus on the light side. What characteristics, emotions, and personality traits do you see in this light person?

Now focus on the dark side, the shadow. What hidden traits, emotions, and characteristics do you see?

Have you previously noticed this shadow? When? Where?

What did you do with your awareness of this person's shadow when you first noticed it?

Did it frighten you? Make you angry? Sad? Did you try to ignore it?

Now that you have seen this person's shadow, how can your relationship grow, change, and become healthier for both of you?

How can you protect yourself from this person's shadow?

Take a long, deep breath, and as you release it, point the crystal down into the ground and allow the person's two sides to come together again.

Once this person is whole, release this image.

Retaining your new, clear vision, and the courage to see with a dark eye, you may open your eyes on the count of ten: one–two–three–four–five–six–seven–eight–nine–ten.

Strengthening Your Aura

✤ *This meditation will assist you in strengthening the energy field around your body, as well as fortifying the life force within you. Gold has always been the substance of alchemical transformation. During the Middle Ages, the alchemist's goal was to turn base metal into gold. If you do this meditation on a regular, even daily, basis, you will find it easier to protect yourself from other people's negative emotions and thoughts, and to ward off the negative energy in your environment.*

Find a comfortable position, either standing or sitting in a straight-backed chair. If you stand, position your feet at shoulder width, slightly bend your knees, and uncross your arms. If you sit, uncross your arms and legs. Close your eyes, take a long, deep breath, and let it out slowly. Allow your breathing to become full, deep, and relaxed.

As you count from ten to zero, allow your rational mind to rest, and you will become more receptive to the wisdom of your soul and its healing power: ten–nine–eight–seven–six–five–four–three–two–one–zero. You are now very deeply relaxed.

Focus your attention far above the top of your head, out into the heavens, and get in touch with a brilliant, powerful, gold light and energy, like the sun flowing down toward you.

Allow yourself to experience this gold light energy flowing all around you and through you, filling your body with its radiance.

With each breath, you inhale this light. As it fills and surrounds you, it gently permeates your entire being and joins the river of life energy already flowing through your body.

Experience this gold light flowing all the way down through your legs and feet, as it connects you with Mother Earth and a sense of secure grounding.

As you fill and strengthen with this gold light energy, you can feel yourself expanding. Your entire aura, your energy field, is becoming bright with gold light and energy, for three feet completely around you, like a golden egg of strength and protection.

With each breath in, you breathe in more power and protection. With each breath out, you release your fears and weaknesses.

Moment by moment you are feeling stronger, more secure, more protected.

All your muscles, nerves, tissues, and organs are being filled and permeated with this gold light. All the cells in your body are beginning to gently vibrate. You can feel the transformation of energy all the way down through your feet and into the ground.

Both your physical body and your aura are becoming stronger as they form a whole system of protection and strength.

As you breathe deeply, you can feel your heart center becoming fortified with love and compassion.

You feel that you can confront any challenges to come your way, and deal with any person you may have to face.

Breathe.

You are radiant with light, love, strength, and energy.

Feel your protection. Feel your internal strength merging with your external protection.

Allow yourself to visualize a situation in which you would like to feel strong and protected.

Feel your new strength, and see yourself able to deal effectively with this situation.

Visualize yourself as able to remain centered, strong, safe, and protected.

As you go out into the external world, you will feel protection from within and all around you. You will feel your radiant aura.

Whenever you feel the need for more energy and protection, you will only have to breathe deeply and focus on allowing the gold light to fill you.

Retaining all of this strength, energy, and protection, you may open your eyes on the count of ten: one–two–three–four–five–six–seven–eight–nine–ten.

Boundaries

✤ *This meditation will help you discover a true sense of healthy boundaries with the world around you. It is a wonderful meditation to do on a daily basis, and can be alternated with "Strengthening Your Aura" whenever you wish.*

Find a comfortable position, either sitting or lying down. Uncross your arms and legs, and close your eyes. Take a long, deep breath, and let it out slowly. Allow your breathing to become full, deep, and relaxed.

As you count from ten to zero, allow your rational mind to rest, and you will become more receptive to the wisdom of your soul and its healing power: ten–nine–eight–seven–six–five–four–three–two–one–zero. You are now very deeply relaxed.

Breathe . . . . . . Allow yourself to feel your breath moving in and out of your body.

Feel this vital, precious air touching the inside of your nose . . . . . . moving down into your bronchial tubes and lungs . . . . . . and becoming one with your body.

Feel where the air meets your physical tissue and becomes your breath.

Allow yourself to feel where your skin meets the air . . . . . . where the air touches your skin.

Feel where your skin touches your clothes . . . . . . and your clothes touch your skin.

Feel your body sitting in the chair . . . . . . and the chair touching your body.

Feel your feet touching the ground . . . . . . and the ground touching your feet.

If you are lying down, feel your body touching the bed . . . . . . and the bed touching your body.

Allow yourself to feel all the ways that you are being touched . . . . . . and all the ways that you are touching.

Allow yourself to become fully conscious where your body's boundaries touch the air . . . . . . your clothes . . . . . . the chair or bed . . . . . . the floor . . . . . . where you touch external reality.

And allow yourself to feel your subtle energy body as it emanates from your body into the space around you.

Allow yourself fully to feel, experience, and be aware of your embodiment.

Retaining this full awareness of your body . . . . . . your breath . . . . . . the air . . . . . . your clothes . . . . . . and all the ways you touch and are touched . . . . . . on the count of ten you may open your eyes: one–two–three–four–five–six–seven–eight–nine–ten.

CHAPTER 4

Creating a New Life

There are moments in all our lives when we realize that we would like to begin again, start our lives anew. Most people think that is impossible, and just keep going along with the way things are, trying to hide their dissatisfaction. As we have seen, trying to repress feelings, memories, and pain only creates deeper wounds that catch up with us later.

To create a new life, we must realize that we cannot do it alone. Human beings in western culture are fond of the old Teutonic ideal of the hero overcoming all odds, slaying the dragon, and winning the golden prize. What this ideal stands for is willpower overcoming all obstacles that stand in its way. What true spirituality is about, and what the eastern religions have helped to teach us, is that the will is our friend and ally insofar as it helps us surrender to the power of the greater mysteries within us. The will is what chooses to surrender to God, Goddess, Higher Power, Spirit—whatever term you feel comfortable using for this spiritual presence.

Christopher Reeve, who played Superman and now struggles with paralysis from a horse jumping accident, stated: "If we can conquer outer space, we can conquer inner space, too." I would change only one word in his statement: Inner space should be explored, honored, meditated upon, and *joined with* as a source of miraculous healing and power. Inner space is our friend, our soul, our source of healing. One does not conquer a friend. One joins forces with it.

Our strength of will can help us choose to create a new life. It can assist us in developing the spiritual discipline to follow through with daily details, such as dream journaling and meditation. It can see us through the difficult times when our faith falters, the world around us falls apart, and our heart is broken. This is a creative use of willpower that can lead to hope, renewal, and resurrection. The word *resurrection* comes from the Latin *resurgere,* meaning to rise again. It does not mean to rise *above,* as the old Teutonic ideal would have us do; but to rise *again* after we have fallen. To rise up from suffering, painful memories, loss of faith and meaning, into a new life of compassion, joy, mystery, acceptance, and courage. Each of us has the opportunity to become resurrected here and now, in each moment. We can choose a new life. We can participate in its creation.

The first meditation, "Not Alone," gives you the opportunity to experience all the ways in which you have tried to control your life and its outcome by the sheer force of your own will. It also gives you the opportunity to change that by asking God to join with you in creating a new life. The next meditation, "Taking Back Your Heart," will allow you to see if you have given your heart away, to whom, and provide you with the opportunity to take it back. To create a new life, a heart of deep passion and love is a necessity.

The next two meditations, "Coping With Change" and "Courage and Commitment," will give you the insight to understand how you tend to resist and defend against change, and how you can develop the courage and commitment to move forward.

"Trusting Your Truth" allows you to reconnect with the place inside you that can see clearly, feel honestly, and know the truth. Most of us have this sensitivity when we are small children, but people and circumstances around us usually invalidate our reality, and then we are left with the realities of other people. This meditation will help you reconnect with your own reality and your inner truth. "Re-Visioning Yourself" will allow you to examine old beliefs and ways that you have of seeing yourself and your life, and then provide you with an opportunity to re-vision your life in a new light.

A new life would not be complete without a deep sense of peace. "Resting in the Heart of God" will allow you to experience this deep peace and connection with God. This is a meditation that you may wish to do on a daily basis. It will bring your mind, heart, and body into wholeness, and give you a resting place. Next to your relationship with yourself, your relationship with God is the most important one in your life.

And finally, "Healing Journey" will allow you to see your healing process as a journey, one that has a past, present, and future. You will be able to examine where you began this journey, how far you have come, and where you would like to arrive in the future. If you have been walking this road with the understanding that healing is a process and also a spiritual discipline, you may be amazed and delighted at the seeds of light that have been planted in your body and soul. Seeds that can grow into full bloom, shine out, and illuminate a world of resurrection and new life.

Not Alone

✤ *This meditation gives you the opportunity to allow God to act as your support and sustenance in creating a new life.*

Find a comfortable position, either sitting or lying down. Uncross your arms and legs, and close your eyes. Take a long, deep breath, and let it out slowly. Allow your breathing to become full, deep, and relaxed.

As you count from ten to zero, allow your rational mind to rest, and you will become more receptive to the wisdom of your soul and its healing power: ten–nine–eight–seven–six–five–four–three–two–one–zero. You are now very deeply relaxed.

Remember all the times in your life when you tried to do something alone, when you felt alone and burdened with doing everything by yourself.

And look at the results.

Remember all the ways in which you tried to give yourself support and sustenance by using something outside you: caffeine, sugar, drugs, cigarettes, alcohol, too much food, too much sleep, too much exercise, too much.

And look at the results.

Remember the times you tried to find all your support and sustenance in another person, all the times you became too dependent upon what they could give you.

And look at the results.

Now, if you can, remember a time when you decided to allow the presence of God to be your support and sustenance. When you decided to stop bargaining for what you wanted and really allow God to be with you.

And look at the results.

Now ask yourself: Am I willing to stop trying to do it alone? Am I willing to admit that I *need* God?

If you are, then ask, right now, for the healing light, presence, and power of God to enter your life and act as your support and sustenance.

Breathe deeply. Image this light, and feel God's presence and power filling your body, heart, and mind.

Visualize what your life can and will be like, from this moment on, supported and sustained by God.

Silently give thanks for God's healing presence in your life.

Retaining this awareness, you may open your eyes on the count of ten: one–two–three–four–five–six–seven–eight–nine–ten.

Taking Back Your Heart

❧ *This meditation will allow you to discover if there was a time in your childhood when you gave away your heart to someone you loved. You will be able to understand why you gave away your heart, what happened to it, and how this affected your life. You will have the opportunity to reclaim your heart and all its love, healing, and passion.*

Find a comfortable position, either sitting or lying down. Uncross your arms and legs, and close your eyes. Take a long, deep breath, and let it out slowly. Allow your breathing to become full, deep, and relaxed.

As you count from ten to zero, allow your rational mind to rest, and you will become more receptive to the wisdom of your soul and its healing power: ten–nine–eight–seven–six–five–four–three–two–one–zero. You are now very deeply relaxed.

Allow your unconscious to give you an image of a time in your childhood when you gave away your heart.

Image this situation as clearly as possible, and feel how you felt then.

How old are you? To whom are you giving your heart? What has led up to this moment?

Feel what happens inside you when you give away your heart.

Is there something you want or need from this other person?

How does the other person respond?

What do they do with your heart?

How has this affected your life?

Tell this person how you feel about them having held your heart.

Feel and image yourself reclaiming your heart.

Repair your heart in whatever ways are necessary.

When your heart is ready, place it in your chest once again.

Feel its presence inside you.

Feel the energy and radiance of your heart flowing to all parts of your body.

Feel its healing power creating new life within you.

Allow yourself to feel the passion, love, hope, and courage that is yours once more.

Feel and see yourself with a new heart, creating a new life of wholeness and healing.

Retaining the full awareness of your heart, you may open your eyes on the count of ten: one–two–three–four–five–six–seven–eight–nine–ten.

Coping with Change

✤ *This meditation will help you examine how you respond when you are threatened by significant change, and begin to provide you with some new and healthy ways to cope.*

Find a comfortable position, either sitting or lying down. Uncross your arms and legs, and close your eyes. Take a long, deep breath, and let it out slowly. Allow your breathing to become full, deep, and relaxed.

As you count from ten to zero, allow your rational mind to rest, and you will become more receptive to the wisdom of your soul and its healing power: ten–nine–eight–seven–six–five–four–three–two–one–zero. You are now very deeply relaxed.

Now focus your attention on your physical body. Notice how it feels now.

Do you notice any places of tension or discomfort? Are there any locations that feel especially relaxed?

Now image yourself in a real situation in which you are threatened by significant change.

Notice how your body responds. Notice your breathing.

How does your physical body respond to the threat of change?

Which parts of your body respond most intensely to this stress?

What are you experiencing in these areas?

Now notice your emotions. What are you feeling?

How is your mind reacting to the threat of this change? What thoughts occur to you?

Now take a long, deep breath, and let it out slowly. Allow your breathing to become full, deep, and relaxed again.

Now focus on your thoughts. What meaning do you give to this change in your life?

How would you have to alter the way you perceive this situation in order to respond differently?

Allow yourself to alter this meaning. If you wish, try to see this change as a life lesson that will deepen and enrich your soul.

Notice how you feel now.

What has happened to your emotional state?

What has happened in your body?

If you have a choice to make about this possible change, how do you perceive your options now?

What decision would you like to make?

Visualize yourself making this decision.

Notice how you feel now.

How is your body responding? Your feelings? Your mind? Your spirit?

Are you responding to this decision in a healthy way?

Are you responding to this possible change in a healthy way?

Feel and visualize yourself responding to the possibility of significant change in a healthy, strong, and open way.

Retaining these healthy responses, you may open your eyes on the count of ten: one–two–three–four–five–six–seven–eight–nine–ten.

Courage and Commitment

✤ *This meditation will assist you in developing courage and making a commitment to your own healing.*

Find a comfortable position, either sitting or lying down. Uncross your arms and legs, and close your eyes. Take a long, deep breath, and let it out slowly. Allow your breathing to become full, deep, and relaxed.

As you count from ten to zero, allow your rational mind to rest, and you will become more receptive to the wisdom of your soul and its healing power: ten–nine–eight–seven–six–five–four–three–two–one–zero. You are now very deeply relaxed.

Image yourself in a situation in which you feel fear. See yourself as clearly as possible and feel how you felt then.

Are you trying to mask or hide your fear? If so, how are you doing this?

Are you feeling that something or someone is the cause of your fear?

Now experiment with courage in the following ways: First, become aware of how much you judge outside forces as being the cause of your fear.

Now take the focus back into yourself, and feel yourself responding in this situation from your core energy, the deepest, most powerful place in your soul.

Breathe . . . . . . Feel and image yourself responding from two places in your body: your solar plexus, your center of willpower; and your heart, your center of love and compassion.

Get in touch with the deepest energy in these two locations, and allow yourself to feel the strength, clarity, security, and compassion that is there. Feel your true life force.

And become aware that your responses begin with you.

Now clear your mind.

Image yourself in a situation in which you feel anger. See yourself as clearly as possible, and feel how you felt then.

Are you trying to mask or hide your anger? If so, how are you doing this?

Are you feeling that something or someone is the cause of your anger?

Now experiment with courage in the following ways: First, become aware of how much you judge outside forces as being the cause of your anger.

Now take the focus back into yourself, and feel yourself responding in this situation from your core energy, the deepest, most powerful place in your soul.

Breathe . . . . . . Feel and image yourself responding from two places in your body: your solar plexus, your center of willpower; and your heart, your center of love and compassion.

Get in touch with the deepest energy in these two locations, and allow yourself to feel the strength, clarity, security, and compassion that is there. Feel your true life force.

And become aware that your responses begin with you.

Now clear your mind.

Image yourself in a situation in which you feel guilt. See yourself as clearly as possible, and feel how you felt then.

Are you trying to mask or hide your guilt? If so, how are you doing this?

Are you feeling that something or someone is the cause of your guilt?

Now experiment with courage in the following ways: First, become aware of how much you judge outside forces as being the cause of your guilt.

Now take the focus back into yourself, and feel yourself responding in this situation from your core energy, the deepest, most powerful place in your soul.

Breathe . . . . . . Feel and image yourself responding from two places in your body: your solar plexus, your center of willpower; and your heart, your center of love and compassion.

Get in touch with the deepest energy in these two locations, and allow yourself to feel the strength, clarity, security, and compassion that is there. Feel your true life force.

And become aware that your responses begin with you.

Now clear your mind.

Image yourself in a situation in which you feel despair. See yourself as clearly as possible, and feel how you felt then.

Are you trying to mask or hide your despair? If so, how are you doing this?

Are you feeling that something or someone is the cause of your despair?

Now experiment with courage in the following ways: First, become aware of how much you judge outside forces as being the cause of your despair.

Now take the focus back into yourself, and feel yourself responding in this situation from your core energy, the deepest, most powerful place in your soul.

Breathe . . . . . . Feel and image yourself responding from two places in your body: your solar plexus, your center of willpower; and your heart, your center of love and compassion.

Get in touch with the deepest energy in these two locations, and allow yourself to feel the strength, clarity, security, and compassion that is there. Feel your true life force.

And become aware that your responses begin with you.

Now clear your mind.

Continue to focus your attention in the middle of your chest and solar plexus. Allow your breathing to help you feel the life force in these centers.

Image yourself standing in front of a white line several feet in front of you on the ground. Gather up all the energy that is inside your heart and will. Breathe.

Feel this life force flowing through the trunk of your body.

Then up into your throat, neck, and head.

Down into your arms and hands.

Down through your legs and feet.

Allow yourself to feel the life force that is your connection to the Earth, the Universe, and to God.

With this energy and courage, make a commitment to your own healing process, and step over the white line in front of you with both feet.

Breathe deeply . . . . . . and allow yourself to experience how it feels to be on the other side of the line.

Staying in touch with your commitment to your healing process, and with all the energy and courage inside, you may open your eyes on the count of ten: one–two–three–four–five–six–seven–eight–nine–ten.

Trusting Your Truth

✦ *This meditation will help you reconnect with your ability to feel, see, and know the truth. It will open that place inside you that has been there since your childhood, when you were in touch with your own reality.*

Find a comfortable position, either sitting or lying down. Uncross your arms and legs, and close your eyes. Take a long, deep breath, and let it out slowly. Allow your breathing to become full, deep, and relaxed.

As you count from ten to zero, allow your rational mind to rest, and you will become more receptive to the wisdom of your soul and its healing power: ten–nine–eight–seven–six–five–four–three–two–one–zero. You are now very deeply relaxed.

Allow yourself to go back to a time in your childhood when you were open, sensitive, aware, and fully alive.

Remember a time when you were aware of the truth; a time when you felt and saw everything clearly and with your heart.

How old are you? How does it feel to see clearly and trust your truth, your sense of reality?

How does your body feel? How does your body know what it knows?

Allow yourself to experience being in love with yourself and the people around you.

Was there a time in your life when it was safe to be in your heart, in love? How does your body experience this love?

Take a long, deep breath, and allow yourself to slowly move forward in your life until you reach a time when you begin to lose touch with this clarity, truth, and love.

What is happening in your life, your family, your environment?

When do you begin to close down or close in? When do you begin to distrust your own feelings, your heart, and your truth?

When do you let someone else's reality become your own?

Notice how your body feels at this age, and even now, as you review this period of your life.

What happens when you shut down your clarity, love, and truth?

Now bring yourself into the present, and take a look at what is going on now in your life.

How much clarity, love, and truth are you experiencing?

How willing are you to once again trust yourself, your heart, and your own truth?

How would your body like to participate in this healing?

Now focus on your heart in the middle of your chest, your center of love and compassion. Begin to breathe in light and energy.

Begin to breathe in a feeling of acceptance—acceptance of what is true.

Allow this acceptance to open your heart and fill it with light and energy.

Allow your heart to open to love. Breathe.

Breathe this light and love into your heart, into your entire body. Notice how your body feels.

For a moment, allow all the people and issues in your life to gently cross your awareness, like clouds in the sky. See them clearly from your heart.

Allow yourself to know the truth about each person and situation. Breathe.

Very slowly and gently, take your hands and place them over your heart, and breathe into your heart.

Allow a feeling of new life, new love, and new clarity to breathe in and out through your heart.

Silently to yourself, repeat the affirmation: "I see and accept the truth."

"With love, I see and accept the truth."

Allow yourself to rest in your heart for a few more minutes. [Two to three minutes.]

Retaining this awareness, allow yourself to open your eyes on the count of ten: one–two–three–four–five–six–seven–eight–nine–ten.

Re-Visioning Yourself

❀ *This meditation will assist you in seeing yourself and your life with new eyes.*

Find a comfortable position, either sitting or lying down. Uncross your arms and legs, and close your eyes. Take a long, deep breath, and let it out slowly. Allow your breathing to become full, deep, and relaxed.

As you count from ten to zero, allow your rational mind to rest, and you will become more receptive to the wisdom of your soul and its healing power: ten–nine–eight–seven–six–five–four–three–two–one–zero. You are now very deeply relaxed.

Allow yourself to become aware of how you see yourself and your life.

Become aware of all the beliefs and ideas that you have.

Is your life what you want it to be? Is it what you hoped and dreamed of?

Are you the person you want to be? Are you who you hoped and dreamed you would become?

Allow yourself to get in touch with your feelings as you examine yourself and your life.

Now allow yourself to go back to the time in your life when you first had this vision of who you wanted to be, and what you wanted your life to become.

What were you like then?

Where did this vision come from? Does it belong to you or to someone else?

Now allow yourself to see all the ways that you have tried to achieve this vision.

Which ways have succeeded?

Which ways have failed?

Are there any aspects of this vision that you need to let go of? Are there any that you need to change?

What kind of *inner* healing would you need to do in order to manifest your true vision in the world?

Breathe.

Allow yourself to drop down into the place inside you that needs healing. Feel the energy that is contained in this deep wound.

Now image this energy as gradually transforming from a dark gray into a shining gold light.

Feel your entire being shining with this golden light of transformation.

Become aware that this energy is now accessible to you for your own healing.

Become aware that as you heal within, so will your life. The strength of this energy will manifest your true vision in the world.

See yourself and your life with new eyes. See yourself living a true life.

Breathe . . . . . . Allow yourself to sit in this energy and vision as long as you wish. When you feel ready, you may open your eyes on the count of ten: one–two–three–four–five–six–seven–eight–nine–ten.

Resting in the Heart of God

❧ *This meditation will take you into a very deep state of peace and union with God. You may wish to pause for a full minute at the end of each line after the countdown.*

Find a comfortable position, either sitting or lying down. Uncross your arms and legs, and close your eyes. Take a long, deep breath, and let it out slowly. Allow your breathing to become full, deep, and relaxed.

As you count down from ten to zero, allow your rational mind to rest, and you will become more receptive to the wisdom of your soul and its healing power: ten—nine—eight—seven—six—five—four—three—two—one—zero. You are now very deeply relaxed.

Allow yourself to continue to drop down, deeper and deeper inside yourself.

Focus on your breath, and feel your breath moving in and out of your chest. With each breath in, drop deeper and deeper.

Breathe in . . . . . . breathe out . . . . . . Allow yourself to breathe in the Breath of God.

Feel your chest and your heart filling with the Breath of God, the Breath of Life.

Allow the awareness of being totally and completely present within your breath, within your body.

Feel the energy of Life gently flowing, through your body, weaving patterns of Creation. Image these patterns as the Light of God.

Deeper and deeper, the Light of God flowing through your body. Allow your body to rest within the Body of God.

Allow your body to rest within the Body of God.

Allow your mind to rest in the presence of this Mystery.

Allow your mind to rest in the Mind of God.

Allow your heart to rest in this peace.

Allow your heart to rest in the Heart of God.

Allow your heart to rest in the Heart of God.

Remaining in this state as long as you wish, you may open your eyes whenever you feel ready to count from one to ten: one–two–three–four–five–six–seven–eight–nine–ten.

Healing Journey

❧ *This meditation will provide you with a way to see your own healing journey. It will allow you to assess how far you have come, what you have learned, and where you would like to go from here.*

Find a comfortable position, either sitting or lying down. Uncross your arms and legs, and close your eyes. Take a long, deep breath, and let it out slowly. Allow your breathing to become full, deep, and relaxed.

As you count from ten to zero, allow your rational mind to rest, and you will become more receptive to the wisdom of your soul and its healing power: ten–nine–eight–seven–six–five–four–three–two–one–zero. You are now very deeply relaxed.

See yourself at the beginning of your healing journey. When and where did this journey begin?

What were you like then?

What were your needs, expectations, and goals?

How much or how little did you know about yourself, your body, and your soul?

Observe how this journey has brought you to the present. (Pause one to two minutes.)

Now take a deep breath. Feel and see yourself in the present. How have you grown? What have you learned about yourself?

Your body?

Your soul?

Your relationship with God?

What are your present needs, expectations, and goals?

Now look into the future. See yourself living a healed life.

What do you see? What are you doing?

How has your healing journey evolved?

See yourself and your new life in a clear way. Let this image stay with you in your heart.

Feel its energy. You are in the process of becoming who you are, deep in your soul.

Allow the past, present, and future to flow together into a healed life.

And allow yourself to trust the healing presence of God in your new life.

Bringing this new vision and trust with you, you may open your eyes on the count of ten: one–two–three–four–five–six–seven–eight–nine–ten.

CHAPTER 5

Helping Others Heal

Intuitive Sensing

Psychometry

Body Scan

Chakra Scan

Laying-on-of-Hands (Basic Form)

Laying-on-of-Hands (Intermediate Form)

Laying-on-of-Hands (Advanced Form)

Distant Healing

Healing the World Soul

*T*here seems to be a deep desire in most of us to ease the suffering of someone we love. Sometimes this desire extends outward to people we hardly know, even to humanity as a whole, as well as to suffering animals, birds, and plants.

The deeper our sense of compassion for our fellow creatures, the more likely it is that we will take the path of becoming a healer. Healers come in many modalities, and it is up to each one of us to find the style that suits us best. Spiritual healing suits me best, and has for twenty years. It is what I teach my students in the TOUCHING SPIRIT® Training Program, a certificate program for people who want to become spiritual healers. The nine meditations and exercises in this chapter are designed to develop your skills as a healer, as well as to further open your intuitive abilities. All the meditations in the first four chapters can be read to others, but these nine are specifically designed to train you to work with other people in a healing capacity. It does not matter if you are a professional healer, an amateur healer, or just a person who cares about helping others. What matters is that you have a heart of deep compassion: This is the only requirement.

There is one other requirement, actually. A true healer is someone who has done, and continues to do, self-healing. If you wish to help others heal, it is vital that you begin with yourself. Thus, I have placed this chapter last, hoping that you would take the time and have the dedication to begin with the earlier chapters. Once your own healing journey is well underway, it is possible to be of assistance to others. It is essential, however, that you remember to continue with your own healing work. Healing is a lifelong practice. There is no finish line. There is no time when you can say "It's done and over! I'm perfect!" If you can accept this, the practice of self-healing can be a rich and rewarding spiritual path. The real treasure of any spiritual path is the journey itself.

There are also many other healing practices that you can use without being a professional healer or health-care professional. You may read certain meditations from earlier chapters to friends and family. If you are a health-care professional, you may wish to integrate these meditations into your existing practice. "Deep Relaxation," "Communicating with Your Body," and "Self-Healing" from chapter 1 make a good trio to use with someone who is physically ill. You would not want to read them all at once, but one at a time, over the period of two or three days. Allow the patient to rest after each meditation and, only when ready, ask the person what they experienced and how they feel. Keep talking to a minimum, as it is good to stay in the deeply relaxed state that the meditations create. It is also important to keep the conversation as positive as possible, since the person is in a very suggestive and open condition after a meditation.

This chapter begins with two exercises to help you develop your intuitive abilities: "Intuitive Sensing" and "Psychometry." The first is a pair-up exercise in which you allow yourself to go into a deeply relaxed and open state, with your rational, thinking mind at rest. In this state, you notice your spontaneous responses to the questions that are asked about the person sitting in front of you. In the second exercise, "Psychometry," you will hold an object that belongs or belonged to someone else, and see how much information you can pick up about that person. Objects, especially metal ones, hold energy. If the object is worn a lot, like a watch or jewelry, or kept on or near the body, like keys, the energy of the person will have imprinted itself in the object. Have you ever noticed how your keys get warm if they are kept in your pocket? That's your energy in the keys.

The gifts of intuition are: *clairsentience, clairvoyance, clairaudience, telepathy,* and *direct knowing.* We have discussed clairsentience in chapter 3, "Psychic Self-Defense." As I mentioned, my natural gift is clairsentience, the ability to feel what other people are feeling, both physically and emotionally. This is what I call being a *psychic sponge.* As I developed clairvoyance, the ability to see information through images and colors, I began to notice that I did not sponge up so much of other people's energies. Being clairvoyant may mean that you can see a scene out of someone's childhood, like a movie, and give the person helpful information that can produce new insights. An example that comes to mind was a woman I worked with many years ago. I saw a rag doll in my inner eye, my third eye. I described this doll to her. She confirmed that she had a doll just like this in her childhood. It had long been forgotten, and she believed the doll had been given away or discarded. This led us into a discussion of her childhood. I don't remember all the details, but I suggested to her that she buy herself a new rag doll and put it on her bed. She resisted. She did not want to feel some unpleasant feelings that were buried in her childhood. Finally, several weeks later, she came in and told me that she had bought a rag doll and placed it on her bed. She was surprised at how many memories came up, and she and I worked through some of the accompanying anger and sadness. Without this clairvoyant image, it may have taken a lot longer to access her memories and accompanying feelings.

There is also something called clairaudience, or clear hearing. Of all the gifts, this tends to be the least understood and, in fact, the Roman Catholic Church tends to believe that only saints and priests have this ability. I disagree. We all have the gift of inner hearing, but we usually ignore it. That little inner voice that says, "Don't park there. You'll get a ticket!" If we ignore the warning, what happens? We get a ticket. Or, in my case, the car was stolen! We can also get this inner information for other people. Sometimes I can hear the person's Higher Self speaking to me when I am doing a body or chakra scan. I'll never forget a beautiful young woman with cancer who came to see me. The first time I did a scan with her, I heard her voice telling me: "You can't heal me. Just love me." She died several months later. I gave her as much love as I could during that difficult period.

Many people think that clairaudience is scary because they are afraid of "hearing voices." We hear our mind talking to us all the time. Sometimes it tells us to pick up the phone and call someone, *now*. Whenever I do this, I usually just catch the person walking in or going out the door. In sessions with patients, that inner voice often has told me what the person needs for healing, such as "no sugar!" When I relay the information, the person sometimes laughs and admits that he or she has been eating too much sugar lately! Often the answer is self-love.

Telepathy, or mind-to-mind communication, is the most common ability. It takes place all day every day and we usually don't realize it. You think of a friend that you haven't seen in a long time, and the phone rings or a letter shows up in the mail an hour later. You wish your husband would bring a pizza home for dinner, and five minutes later he walks in with a pizza. These examples take place in healing as well. Sometimes people are afraid to tell me certain details of their lives. If the person is holding the thought in mind, it often gets relayed to me, and I pick it up clairaudiently or clairvoyantly. Examples might be smoking, alcoholism, sexual abuse, or violence. These things are often hard to talk about with a stranger. If I get the information telepathically, I can often find a gentle way to encourage the person to tell me about it, without having to bring it up. It is absolutely essential, when doing intuitive work, that you *never* suggest to someone that they were sexually abused, and *never* diagnose a medical condition. If you feel that someone has such a problem, it is wiser to suggest that they consult a psychotherapist or a physician.

The most comprehensive ability is direct knowing. You just know something. You are not sure how you know it, but you do. The old romantic notion of seeing someone across a crowded room and knowing that he or she is meant for you is a good example. Or maybe it is an apartment or house. I remember walking into my first apartment in New York City. I had been to see about a dozen places, none of them right. When I walked into this one, I knew as soon as I stepped through the door that this was the one. Sometimes when students show up in workshops, I know which ones are going to follow through and which ones are going to drop out. I'm sure you have your own examples. Direct knowing seems to take place when all the intuitive gifts come together at once, so quickly, in such an integrated way, that we just *know.* There is no doubt, no questioning. We just know what is true. It is true knowing.

These are the four rules of intuitive work: 1) take what you get; 2) don't edit; 3) don't judge; and 4) always assume it's not yours, until proven otherwise.

Rule 1. Take what you get. This means that when you get a piece of information, accept it. Don't throw it away because you don't like it, don't understand it, or think it's irrelevant. If you "see" a slimy green snake as your partner's pet, take what you get! You may be right!

Rule 2. Don't edit. This means that you should accept the information as it comes to you without changing it in any way. If you "hear" your partner's father screaming curse words in rage, don't edit out the curse words. They may be the most important and validating part of the information.

Rule 3. Don't judge. This means two things: don't judge what you get as stupid, silly, or wrong; and, it means don't judge your partner or anything that you learn about your partner.

Rule 4. Always assume it's not yours until proven otherwise. This means that you should assume the information belongs to your partner, not to you. For example, if you "feel" that your partner's greatest fear is abandonment, and that is also your greatest fear, don't assume you are overlaying your own fear onto your partner. Just because it is also your fear, doesn't mean it is not your partner's! What's the old saying? Just because you're paranoid doesn't mean someone isn't after you!

These are the best four rules to use when attempting to develop your intuitive abilities. A few precautions are: Do *not* diagnose any physical ailments by using the name of a disease. If you feel an area is unhealthy, suggest that your partner see a physician. Do *not* prescribe medications, foods, or treatments. And *never* suggest to someone that they have been sexually abused.

If you have used "Intuitive Sensing" and "Psychometry," and discovered that you are very intuitive, or if you are a teacher who works with groups of healers, you may wish to try some of the scanning exercises, such as "Body Scan" and "Chakra Scan." These exercises will train your hands to pick up subtle shifts in energy coming from other people's bodies. The following list is a guide to possible ways to interpret what you feel. The most important factor is your own intuition. If this chart and your intuition disagree, trust your intuiton and get validation from the person you are scanning, another healer, or a teacher of healing.

Your hands feel:
- Gentle warmth: healthy energy
- Cold: lack of energy flow
- Cold and expansion or movement: high level of psychic openness or lack of boundaries
- Pleasant tingling: healthy energy flow
- Unpleasant tingling or prickling: imbalance or pain
- Vibration or pulsing: energized
- Nothing: a "dead" spot, no energy
- Magnetic pull toward body: energy needed
- Magnetic push away from body: good energy flow or resistance
- A "wall," hands stop and don't move: blockage, resistance
- Pain, pressure: inflammation, pain, illness
- Extreme heat: inflammation or illness
- Contraction and heat: tension
- Slight shaking: energy flowing
- Violent shaking: imbalance, pain, or illness being discharged

The energy scans will also train you to pay attention to all the impressions, images, colors, words, and feelings that are happening in your own body and mind as your hands are doing the scanning. You learn to use your hands as dowsing rods, and yourself as a barometer. "Body Scan" will focus on your hands scanning through the physical body of your partner, whereas "Chakra Scan" will focus your hands on the subtle energies coming from your partner's seven major chakras.

Again, it is very important to remember that, no matter how intuitive and accurate you are, unless you are a medical doctor, you should never attempt to diagnose another person's medical condition. Besides being against the law, you could be wrong. This could be detrimental to the other's person's health, and could cause the person to postpone seeking needed medical attention. These exercises are for educational purposes only. If you have questions about something that you have felt in another person's body, you should speak with a health-care professional, and suggest to the person you are working with that he or she consult a physician.

Once you have developed your intuitive sensitivities, you can participate in someone's healing by doing "Laying-on-of-Hands." Begin with the basic form, which focuses on one location of the body and lasts about twenty minutes. This process creates an imprint of energy that catalyzes healing in the body. It helps the body mobilize its own natural healing responses. All mothers who touch their children with love and comfort are doing a laying-on-of-hands. In fact, this basic form of laying-on-of-hands can be used to heal children and animals. I once sent it to a woman whose dog was aging and developing paralysis in its hind legs. The dog could no longer walk. She wrote me back several weeks later that her dog was jumping around like a puppy again. Animals and children do not have the complex thought patterns and belief systems that adults have. They can more easily allow the healing energy to do its work with no interference from their minds. The most important factor is the love that is felt deep in your heart as you are giving the healing. The love gets transmitted with the energy, and it is really love that is the most powerful healer of all.

If you are an experienced healer or bodyworker, you may wish to use the intermediate or advanced form of laying-on-of-hands. The intermediate form has you begin at the head, move to the location that needs healing, and then end at the feet, on both sides of the body. This version takes about thirty minutes. The advanced form has you work on both sides of the body as well, but adds all the locations of the chakras. This version takes about forty-five minutes, and should only be attempted if you are experienced.

It is always essential that you receive someone's permission to touch them. The laying-on-of-hands can be done several inches above the body if someone is uncomfortable with direct touch. It is vital that you do not touch the face, eyes, throat, breasts, pelvis, groin, or pubic area. These locations are particularly sensitive for most people, and associated with intimacy. The person will feel the healing energy even if your hands are several inches away. Make sure to tell the person that if, at any time, they want you to remove your hands or stop the healing, they should let you know and you will do so immediately.

It is important that you be in relatively good health if you wish to do healing through the laying-on-of-hands. If you have a cold, flu, or sore throat, you could transmit these germs to the patient. If you have a headache, the person could pick up that as well. If you have a back problem, your back could potentially feel worse after holding your hands over someone for half an hour. If you are a patient with a serious illness, like cancer or AIDS, it would be better if you prayed for the person, and let someone else do the physical healing work. When your own body is in need of healing, it cannot transfer properly the healing energy to someone else. It is also vital that, if your hands are cold, you keep them above the body. Wait until your hands warm before you actually touch someone.

The person receiving the healing must be completely comfortable, and preferably lying down on a massage table or a bed. You can use the bed of the person on whom you are working, but never use your own bed. If need be, you may use a chair. It is good to clear the space before and after a healing. You want to make sure that the healing room is as neutral as possible, meaning that it is free from other energies and influences. Turn off the phone, television, and radio. Put a sign on the door so that no one rings the doorbell. Take out any clocks that are ticking. Take off your watch and any jewelry that you have on your body. Any kind of metal will effect the flow of healing energy, so you need to have the patient also remove his or her jewelry. Place these pieces of jewelry in another room. Then light a candle and burn some incense or sage. Fire and powerful herbs and oils have been used for thousands of years in healing rituals. They help set the energy and ambiance of a room. If you wish, you may play some soft and slow music in the background. It is vital that the music be low, barely audible, since as the room quiets down and you begin the healing, the music will seem louder than when you first put it on. Use an autoreverse player for cassette tapes, or a CD that keeps playing, since you don't want it to stop or click off in the middle of your healing.

It is good if the person falls asleep during and/or after the healing, since a deeply relaxed body is one that can best mobilize its healing energies. Let the person sleep as long as possible. Upon awakening, the person may feel refreshed or, more likely, very groggy at first. Gently help the person off the table or out of bed; get a glass of water for them. Don't be surprised if it takes them a long time to fully "come back." Such deep relaxation is rare in today's fast-paced world. It is a luxury that should be more common. If possible, suggest that the person take it easy for the rest of the day, walk and talk slowly, eat well, and treat themselves with care. Again, not too much talking after a laying-on-of-hands.

At the end of the healing, after the person has left the room, relight the sage or incense, open the windows, and walk around the room in a circle with the scent. This will help release any energies that have been in the room. Also wave the sage over the table, bed, or chair. If you wish, you may take a small bowl of water, say a prayer of cleansing over it, and sprinkle it around the room. An appropriate prayer might be: "May the water clear this room, leaving it filled only with love."

Prayer is one of the most powerful techniques that we can use to help ourselves and others. As recent scientific studies and books have shown, prayer is one of the most effective spiritual practices in existence, and has been used by almost all religions and cultures around the world. Even western physicians with conventional medical practices have begun to pray with their patients.

"Distant Healing" provides a way for you to focus on a person's face and body, or name, as a way to send healing to someone who is not in your presence. It takes what we think of as prayer, and adds guided imagery to it. In this way, we are using the right side of the brain in conjunction with the left side, to create a more powerful response within us. You can ask permission of the person to whom you wish to send healing. I have found over the years, however, that most people are happy to receive healing. If the person does not want to let in the healing energy that you are sending them, it will bounce off.

The final meditation, "Healing the World Soul," is a lovely way for you to participate in healing at a collective and universal level. We all wish for peace on earth, and for a universe that is full of love and harmony. By opening your own heart and sending this energy out through the entire universe, you can do your part in helping to heal the world soul.

With a little care, you may find that you fall in love with healing as your spiritual path. If you do, seek out a teacher who can help you on your journey. Allow yourself to be guided by your deep inner knowing as well as by careful common sense. Make sure that the person you pick as your teacher is dedicated to self-healing as his or her spiritual path. As you heal from within, you will become a healer who can help others heal. Most important, your presence will be healing.

Intuitive Sensing

✤ *This meditation will assist you in opening your gifts of intuition:
clairsentience, clairvoyance, clairaudience, telepathy, and direct knowing. You need a partner for this exercise. One person remains passive;
the other is active. After sharing and a short break, you can reverse roles.
Pay attention to the wrong answers as carefully as you do to the right
answers. They may teach you something about how you receive and
process information. Remember the four rules of intuitive work: 1) take
what you get; 2) don't edit; 3) don't judge; and 4) always assume it's not
yours (meaning: the information belongs to your partner)!*

There are a few cautions: Do not *diagnose any physical ailments by
using the name of a disease. If you feel an area is unhealthy, suggest that
your partner see a physician. Do not prescribe medications, foods, or
treatments. And* never *suggest to someone that they have been sexually
abused.*

Place two chairs across from each other, so that you and your partner
can sit facing each other without touching.

Make sure you have chosen which partner is going to be active and
which partner is going to be passive. Both of you should begin by
closing your eyes. When you open your eyes, the passive partner
may look aside or down, but must keep their eyes open.

Close your eyes. Take a long, deep breath, and let it out slowly. As
you count from ten to zero, allow your rational mind to take a
rest and your body to relax: ten—nine—eight—seven—six—five—four—
three—two—one—zero.

If you are active, allow yourself to get in touch with a bright, white
light in the heavens. See and feel it flowing down toward you and
all around you.

As you do, breathe this light into your body. Feel it entering your lungs, and filling your body with light.

Experience this light energy freely flowing in and out of each chakra, and easily up and down your spine.

At the base of your spine, your first chakra of grounding and security, see and feel this white light gently moving in a circular motion.

Allow it to travel down through your legs and into the ground, connecting you with Mother Earth.

Feel the energy flowing easily up and down your legs.

Now allow the energy to flow gently in a spiral motion from your first chakra into your second, in your pelvis, your center of clairsentience, clear feeling.

And into your third chakra in your solar plexus. Allow your center of will to relax.

And into your heart chakra in the middle of your chest, your center of compassion. Breathe.

And into your throat chakra, your center of clairaudience, clear hearing.

And into your third eye between your eyebrows, your center of clairvoyance, clear seeing; and telepathy, mind-to-mind communication.

And up to the crown chakra at the top of your head, your center of direct knowing.

Feel the energy flowing easily through all your chakras.

Now focus your attention on your third eye between your eyebrows. Allow yourself to feel the energy flowing gently in a circular motion, opening your center of psychic sight.

Very slowly open your eyes and look at and around your partner's face and head. What do you see? What is the first thing you notice?

In meeting this person for the first time, what would you notice?

Do you see any light, movement, or energy around your partner's head?

Now look more deeply into your partner's face. Who is this person sitting in front of you?

What emotions do you see, present and past?

What was this person like as a child? Drop all thinking and just see, feel, sense, and hear.

What was this person's mother like?

Does your partner have any of her characteristics?

Is she still alive?

What was this person's father like?

Does your partner have any of his characteristics?

Is he still alive?

Did your partner have any pets as a child? What kind?

Do you hear any names?

Does your partner have any pets now? What kind?

Do you hear any names?

What is your partner's greatest fear?

What is your partner's greatest gift?

Does your partner need to forgive someone? Who?

What is the most important lesson your partner can learn in this life?

Now allow your attention to focus just above the top of your partner's head. Imagine a ball of white light gently moving down through your partner's head and body, illuminating any areas that need attention or healing. (Pause one to two minutes.)

Breathe. Drop all thinking and just see, feel, hear, and know. (Pause one to two minutes.)

Now place your awareness at your partner's feet. On the count of three the white light will focus, like a laser beam, on the area of your partner's body that needs the most healing: one–two–three.

Focus your attention here. Breathe. What do you sense?

What do you feel?

What do you see?

What do you hear?

What do you seem to know about this area of your partner's body?

What is needed for healing to take place?

On the count of three you will get a spontaneous image of a healing symbol: one–two–three. Accept what you see, even if its meaning is unclear.

Image your partner completely whole, healed, and full of energy.

Close your eyes. Take a long, deep breath, and let it out slowly. When you open your eyes, tell your partner what you have felt, seen, and heard. Allow the information to flow in the order it comes, and when you are finished, let your partner respond. You may open your eyes on the count of ten: one–two–three–four–five–six–seven–eight–nine–ten.

Remember: Do *not* diagnose any physical ailments by using the name of a disease. If you feel an area is unhealthy, suggest that your partner see a physician. Do *not* prescribe medications, foods, or treatments. And *never* suggest to someone that they have been sexually abused.

When you are finished relating your impressions, wash your hands in cold water, and sit down to clear with the following exercise: Take a long, deep breath, and let it out slowly. Feel and image any energy that you have absorbed from the person as being released up and out the top of your head. Start at the bottom of your feet, move all the way up through the trunk of your body, and then release it out of the top of your head. When you feel completely cleared, you may open your eyes.

Psychometry

❖ *This exercise is a fun and easy way to increase your intuitive sensitivities. You may do it alone with objects from people you know, or with a partner. Having a partner gives you immediate feedback, which is essential to learning whether you are right or wrong. After a short break, you may then reverse roles. Using objects that belong only to one person, such as a watch, keys, or a piece of jewelry, will be easier, but you may use objects handed down through family members, relatives, and friends. In this case, you may pick up information both about your partner and the person who gave it to your partner.*

Place two chairs across from each other, so that you and your partner may sit facing each other closely but without touching.

Choose your roles. One of you will be doing the exercise, and the other will offer an object. Only the object that will be used immediately should be in the room. For the moment, place it aside but within reach. Leave any other objects in another room.

Uncross your arms and legs, and close your eyes. Take a long, deep breath, and let it out slowly. Allow your breathing to become full, deep, and relaxed.

As you count from ten to zero, allow your rational mind to rest, and you will become more receptive to the wisdom of your soul and its deep intuition: ten–nine–eight–seven–six–five–four–three–two–one–zero. You are now very deeply relaxed.

Focus your attention far above the top of your head, out into the heavens, and get in touch with a very brilliant, powerful, white light coming down to you in a stream of energy.

Allow this white light to flow all around you and, with each breath, allow it flow into your lungs and through your entire body.

Experience this light energy freely flowing in and out of each chakra, and easily up and down your spine.

At the base of your spine, your first chakra of grounding and security, see and feel this white light gently moving in a circular motion.

As it does, allow it to travel down through your legs and into the ground, connecting you with Mother Earth.

Feel the energy flowing easily up and down your legs.

Now allow the energy to flow gently in a spiral motion from your first chakra into your second, in your pelvis, your center of clairsentience, clear feeling.

And into your third chakra in your solar plexus. Allow your center of willpower to relax.

And into your heart chakra in the middle of your chest, your center of compassion. Breathe.

And into your throat chakra, your center of clairaudience, clear hearing.

And into your third eye between your eyebrows, your center of clairvoyance, clear seeing; and telepathy, mind-to-mind communication.

And up to the crown chakra at the top your head, your center of direct knowing.

Feel the energy flowing easily through all your chakras.

Now focus your attention on your third eye between your eyebrows. Allow yourself to feel the energy flowing gently in a circular motion, opening your center of psychic sight.

Change your focus to your hands. With both hands lying on your legs, palms up, feel the chakras of energy in the centers of your palms.

As these chakras open, feel the flow of energy and sensitivity down into your fingers and fingertips.

Your hands are now like dowsing rods: sensitive, open, and ready to receive impressions.

Take the object from your partner.

As you feel this object in your hands, what is your first impression?

What physical sensations do you feel in your hands as you hold it?

Keeping your eyes closed, can you tell what it is?

Drop all thinking and just feel, sense, see, hear, and know.

How old is this object?

To whom does it belong?

Was it a gift? Or bought by the person for personal use?

How many owners has it had?

Now take a long, deep breath, and allow yourself to drop down even more deeply.

How does your body feel as you are holding this object?

What emotions do you feel?

Do you hear any words? Phrases?

Do you see any colors?

Do you see any images?

Allow these images to unfold like movie scenes in your mind.

Drop all thinking, and just follow where the images take you.

Is there anything else you pick up from this object?

When you open your eyes, you will be able to tell your partner the impressions that you have received from this object. On the count of ten you may open your eyes: one–two–three–four–five–six–seven–eight–nine–ten.

When you are finished relating your impressions, hand the object back to your partner, wash your hands in cool water, and sit down to clear with the following exercise: Take a long, deep breath, and let it out slowly. Feel and image any energy that you have absorbed from the object as being released up and out the top of your head. Start at the bottom of your feet, move all the way up through the trunk of your body, and then release it out the top of your head. When you feel completely cleared, you may open your eyes.

Body Scan

✤ *This exercise will teach you how to sensitize your hands and use them to scan the energy emanations coming from another person's body. You need two chairs, preferably without arms, and a partner. You may wish to keep a pencil and paper on a table by your side, so that you can jot down any notes as you are doing the scan. This exercise will take about thirty minutes for each person's turn.*

Place two chairs across from each other, so that you and your partner may sit facing each other closely but without touching.

Choose your roles. One of you will be doing the scan, and the other will be passive.

You should both begin by sitting. Initially, you will be taken through a brief chakra-opening that will increase your intuitive sensitivity. After this, the scanner will stand behind the partner's chair. Halfway through the scan, the scanner will sit and the partner will stand. You will be told when to switch positions.

Uncross your arms and legs, and close your eyes. Take a long, deep breath, and let it out slowly. Allow your breathing to become full, deep, and relaxed.

As you count from ten to zero, allow your rational mind to rest, and you will become more receptive to the wisdom of your unconscious and its deep intuition: ten–nine–eight–seven–six–five–four–three–two–one–zero. You are now very deeply relaxed.

Focus your attention far above the top of your head, out into the heavens, and get in touch with a very brilliant, powerful, white light coming down to you in a stream of energy.

Allow this white light to flow all around you and, with each breath, allow it to flow into your lungs and through your entire body.

Experience this light energy freely flowing in and out of each chakra, and easily up and down your spine.

At the base of your spine, your first chakra of grounding and security, see and feel this white light gently moving in a circular motion.

As it does, allow it to travel down through your legs and into the ground, connecting you with Mother Earth.

Feel the energy flowing easily up and down your legs.

Now allow the energy to flow gently in a spiral motion from your first chakra into your second, in your pelvis, your center of clairsentience, clear feeling.

And into your third chakra in your solar plexus. Allow your center of will to relax.

And into your heart chakra in the middle of your chest, your center of compassion. Breathe.

And into your throat chakra, your center of clairaudience, clear hearing.

And into your third eye between your eyebrows, your center of clairvoyance, clear seeing; and telepathy, mind-to-mind communication.

And up to the crown chakra at the top of your head, your center of direct knowing.

Feel the energy flowing easily through all your chakras.

Now focus your attention on your third eye between your eyebrows. Allow yourself to feel the energy flowing gently in a circular motion, opening your center of psychic sight.

Change your focus to your hands. With both hands lying on your legs, palms up, feel the chakras of energy in the centers of your palms.

As these chakras open, feel the flow of energy and sensitivity down into your fingers and fingertips.

Your hands are now like dowsing rods: sensitive, open, and ready to receive impressions.

At this point, stand behind your partner's chair to begin the scan. With your knees slightly bent and your body relaxed, close your eyes and breath deeply.

Raise your arms as high as you can. Keep your eyes closed and your hands and fingers relaxed, and lower your arms so your hands come down over your partner's shoulders. As soon as you feel any kind of subtle energy coming from your partner's shoulders, stop there.

Hold your hands above your partner's shoulders, and allow yourself to tune into the energies emanating from both shoulders.

Do you notice any difference between the right and left shoulders?

Is one of your hands higher than the other?

Do you feel any discomfort, tingling, prickling, heat, or cold?

Is the energy comfortable and flowing easily, or is it uncomfortable and blocked?

Take a moment to make any notes you wish.

Now move around to the side of your partner's chair. If you are right-handed, you may wish to stand on the right; if left-handed, on the left.

Place your hands side by side above the top of your partner's head, as high as you can. Keeping your palms and fingers relaxed, lower your hands slowly, until you can feel energy emanating from your partner's head.

Now slowly move your hands down, so that one hand moves in back of the head and the other in front of the sinuses and eyes. Allow your hands to gently move across these areas, paying attention to everything you see, feel, and hear.

Allow yourself to trust your impressions. Do you notice any areas that feel different? Disturbed? Warm or cold? Do any areas make your hands hurt?

Continue to allow your hands to descend through your partner's ears, teeth, jaw, neck, and throat.

Take a moment to makes any notes you wish.

Now let your hands descend through your partner's chest, heart and lungs, as well as upper back and spine.

Next move down through the shoulders, arms, and hands.

Allow yourself to trust your impressions. Do you notice any areas that feel different? Disturbed? Warm or cold? Do any areas make your hands hurt?

Take a moment to makes any notes you wish.

At this point, ask your partner to stand sideways to your chair while you sit. Suggest that they bend their legs slightly and close their eyes.

Now place your hands one in front of the stomach and the other at the midback. Use your hands to scan through these areas, as well as the liver and gall bladder under the right rib, the spleen and pancreas under the left rib, and the kidneys and adrenal glands at the back of the waist.

Allow yourself to trust your impressions. Do you notice any areas that feel different? Disturbed? Warm or cold? Do any areas make your hands hurt?

Take a moment to make any notes you wish.

Allow your hands to scan through the pelvis and reproductive organs, the intestines, colon, hips, and lower back.

Allow yourself to trust your impressions. Do you notice any areas that feel different? Disturbed? Warm or cold? Do any areas make your hands hurt?

Take a moment to make any notes you wish.

Go all the way down the legs, knees, ankles, and feet.

Allow yourself to trust your impressions. Do you notice any areas that feel different? Disturbed? Warm or cold? Do any areas make your hands hurt?

Take a moment to make any notes you wish.

If there is any area of your partner's body that you would like to rescan, take a minute and do that now.

When you are finished, tell your partner that they may sit, and take a seat yourself as well. Close your eyes, and allow yourself to completely relax.

You may now wash your hands in cold water, and get your partner and yourself a glass of room-temperature water.

When you come back, you may go over your notes with your partner.

Remember: Do *not* diagnose any physical ailments by using the name of a disease. If you feel an area is unhealthy, suggest that your partner see a physician. Do *not* prescribe medications, foods, or treatments. And *never* suggest to someone that they have been sexually abused.

Chakra Scan

❧ *This exercise will teach you how to sensitize your hands and use them to scan the energy emanations coming from another person's seven major chakras. As the scanner, you will be taken through a brief chakra opening of your own in order to increase your sensitivity. You need two chairs, preferably without arms, and a partner. You may wish to keep a pencil and paper on a table by your side, so that you can jot down any notes as you are doing the scan. This exercise will take about forty-five minutes for each person's turn.*

Place two chairs across from each other, so that you and your partner may sit facing each other closely but without touching.

Choose your roles. One of you will be doing the scan, and the other will be passive.

You should both begin by sitting. The scanner will be taken through a brief opening before the partner scan. When the partner scan begins, the scanner will begin by sitting next to the partner, who will be standing sideways. Halfway through the scan, the scanner will stand and the partner will sit. You will be told when to switch positions.

Uncross your arms and legs, and close your eyes. Take a long, deep breath, and let it out slowly. Allow your breathing to become full, deep, and relaxed.

As you count from ten to zero, allow your rational mind to rest, and you will become more receptive to the wisdom of your soul and its deep intuition: ten–nine–eight–seven–six–five–four–three– two–one–zero. You are now very deeply relaxed.

Focus your attention far above the top of your head, out into the heavens, and get in touch with a very brilliant, powerful, white light coming down to you in a stream of energy.

Allow this white light to flow all around you and, with each breath, allow it to flow into your lungs and through your entire body.

Experience this light energy freely flowing in and out of each chakra, and easily up and down your spine.

At the base of your spine, your first chakra of grounding and security, see and feel this white light gently moving in a circular motion.

As it does, allow it to travel down through your legs and into the ground, connecting you with Mother Earth.

Feel the energy flowing easily up and down your legs.

Now allow the energy to flow gently in a spiral motion from your first chakra into your second, in your pelvis, your center of clairsentience, clear feeling.

And into your third chakra in your solar plexus. Allow your center of will to relax.

And into your heart chakra in the middle of your chest, your center of compassion. Breathe.

And into your throat chakra, your center of clairaudience, clear hearing.

And into your third eye between your eyebrows, your center of clairvoyance, clear seeing; and telepathy, mind-to-mind communication.

And up to the crown chakra at the top of your head, your center of direct knowing.

Feel the energy flowing easily through all your chakras.

Now focus your attention on your third eye between your eyebrows. Allow yourself to feel the energy flowing gently in a circular motion, opening your center of psychic sight.

Change your focus to your hands. With both hands lying on your legs, palms up, feel the chakras of energy in the centers of your palms.

As these chakras open, feel the flow of energy and sensitivity down into your fingers and fingertips.

Your hands are now like dowsing rods: sensitive, open, and ready to receive impressions.

At this point the person being scanned should stand, move the chair out of the way, and stand sideways to the scanner, who is sitting.

Beginning with your hands at the base of your partner's spine, one hand in front and the other in back, move your hands as far apart as you can. Keeping your shoulders and hands relaxed, very slowly move your hands into the body, until you can begin to feel a subtle energy emanating from your partner's first chakra, the center of security.

Hold your hands here and allow yourself to feel the energy with your hands. Is the energy warm or cool? Still or moving? Comfortable or uncomfortable?

Is your partner holding the energy close to the body, or is it expansive?

Do you see any color?

Hear any words or phrases?

See any images?

Sense any emotions?

Take a moment and write down any impressions you wish. (Pause one to two minutes, as necessary.)

Now move up to the second chakra, the center of sexuality and creative life force. With your hands as far apart as possible, place one hand in front of the pelvis, and the other in back of the sacrum, or lower back.

Hold your hands here and allow yourself to feel the energy with your hands. Is the energy warm or cool? Still or moving? Comfortable or uncomfortable?

Is your partner holding the energy close to the body, or is it expansive?

Do you see any color?

Hear any words or phrases?

See any images?

Sense any emotions?

Take a moment and write down any impressions you wish. (Pause one to two minutes, as necessary.)

Now move up to the third chakra, the center of willpower, motivation, and vitality. With your hands as far apart as possible, place one hand in front of the solar plexis, and the other in the center of the back.

Hold your hands here and allow yourself to feel the energy with your hands. Is the energy warm or cool? Still or moving? Comfortable or uncomfortable?

Is your partner holding the energy close to the body, or is it expansive?

Do you see any color?

Hear any words or phrases?

See any images?

Sense any emotions?

Take a moment and write down any impressions you wish. (Pause one to two minutes, as necessary.)

At this point the person being scanned may sit down, and the scanner should stand and move their chair aside.

Now move up to the fourth chakra, the center of love and compassion. With your hands as far apart as possible, place one hand in front of the chest, and the other in the center of the upper back.

Hold your hands here and allow yourself to feel the energy with your hands. Is the energy warm or cool? Still or moving? Comfortable or uncomfortable?

Is your partner holding the energy close to the body, or is it expansive?

Do you see any color?

Hear any words or phrases?

See any images?

Sense any emotions?

Take a moment and write down any impressions you wish. (Pause one to two minutes, as necessary.)

Now move up to the fifth chakra, the center of self-expression. With your hands as far apart as possible, place one hand in front of the throat, and the other at the back of the neck.

Hold your hands here and allow yourself to feel the energy with your hands. Is the energy warm or cool? Still or moving? Comfortable or uncomfortable?

Is your partner holding the energy close to the body, or is it expansive?

Do you see any color?

Hear any words or phrases?

See any images?

Sense any emotions?

Take a moment and write down any impressions you wish. (Pause one to two minutes, as necessary.)

Now move up to the sixth chakra, the center of clear vision and intuition. With your hands as far apart as possible, place one hand in front of the forehead, and the other at the back of the head.

Hold your hands here and allow yourself to feel the energy with your hands. Is the energy warm or cool? Still or moving? Comfortable or uncomfortable?

Is your partner holding the energy close to the body, or is it expansive?

Do you see any color?

Hear any words or phrases?

See any images?

Sense any emotions?

Take a moment and write down any impressions you wish. (Pause one to two minutes, as necessary.)

Now move up to the seventh chakra, the center of spiritual consciousness. With your hands as high as possible, place both hands side by side above the head.

Hold your hands here and allow yourself to feel the energy with your hands. Is the energy warm or cool? Still or moving? Comfortable or uncomfortable?

Is your partner holding the energy close to the body, or is it expansive?

Do you see any color?

Hear any words or phrases?

See any images?

Sense any emotions?

Take a moment and write down any impressions you wish. (Pause one to two minutes, as necessary.)

If you wish, you may take a minute to rescan any chakra. (Pause one minute.)

When you are finished, take a seat. Close your eyes and allow yourself to completely relax.

You may now wash your hands in cold water, and get yourself and your partner a glass of room-temperature water.

When you come back, you may go over your notes with your partner.

Remember: Do *not* diagnose any physical ailments by using the name of a disease. If you feel an area is unhealthy, suggest that your partner see a physician. Do *not* prescribe medications, foods, or treatments. And *never* suggest to someone that they have been sexually abused.

Laying-on-of-Hands
(Basic Form)

✤ *This meditation will guide you through a basic form of the laying-on-of-hands. It can be used with adults, children, and animals. To begin, place the person or animal in a comfortable position either sitting or lying down—they can even be asleep. Position yourself so that you will be able to rest your hands either above or lightly on the afflicted area. Make sure you are in a position that will be comfortable for you to hold for about twenty minutes. If you become uncomfortable at any time, raise your hands, change your position, and replace your hands. Remember to breathe!*

If you are being healed, take your position in the chair, or on the table or bed. Take a long, deep breath and relax, consciously setting your intention to open and be receptive to the healing you are about to receive.

If you are the healer, begin with your arms at your sides, take a deep breath, and close your eyes. Allow your breathing to become full, deep, and relaxed.

Begin with a prayer that is simple and appropriate for your spiritual beliefs, such as: I ask that my ego be put aside and that this healing be for the highest good of the person (or animal) receiving it. I ask for God's healing love and power to be present.

As you count from ten to zero, allow your rational mind to rest and become even more deeply relaxed: ten–nine–eight–seven–six–five–four–three–two–one–zero. Breathe. You are now very deeply relaxed.

Focus your attention far above the top of your head, out into the heavens, and get in touch with a brilliant, powerful, white light and energy flowing down toward you.

Allow yourself to experience this light energy flowing all around you and through you, filling your body with its radiance.

With each breath, you inhale this light. As it fills and surrounds you, it gently permeates your entire being and joins the river of life energy already flowing through your body.

Focus your attention on your heart chakra in the middle of your chest, your center of love and compassion. Visualize the white light concentrating its energy here, and begin to feel it moving in a gentle, slow, and circular motion.

As it flows, it begins to open your heart center. Breathe deeply and allow your chest to open fully, making room for this light energy.

As you do, you can feel the love and compassion in your heart opening for the person in front of you. The love and light energy combine into a powerful healing energy.

As this healing energy becomes stronger and fuller, it moves up into your shoulders, down your arms, and into your hands. You may begin to feel a tingling, pulsation, or even warmth, in your palms and fingers.

Now lift your arms and place both of your hands palm to palm in front of you, about ten to twelve inches apart. Keep your hands and fingers relaxed, move them slightly toward and away from each other. You will begin to feel the sense of energy between them, almost like a gentle magnetic pull.

Now lift your arms and place both of your hands, palms down, about three feet above the body of the person in front of you. Focus on the area that needs healing. If they are sitting in a chair, you can place one hand in front and the other in back of the body.

Close your eyes again and allow yourself to begin to feel the energy from your hands meeting the energy emanating from the body.

If this person is in pain or discomfort, or has some kind of infection or inflammation, you may feel this in your hands. To clear their energy field, gently move your hands in a sweeping or brushing motion above the body.

If your hands become uncomfortable or painful at any time, remove them and shake them gently away from you. Replace them slightly higher or farther away than they were previously placed.

Healing is usually pleasant and comforting, but if the person, child, or animal experiences any kind of agitation or discomfort as you place your hands over their body, remove them and replace them several inches farther away.

Wait patiently as the healing energy begins to flow.

You may notice that your hands begin to lower or move closer on their own, as the healing is received. You may even find that you can lightly rest your hands on the body.

Drop all thinking and breathe easily and gently.

Focus all your attention on your hands, allowing the healing energy to flow though you.

See the receiver as whole and healthy.

Feel the love and energy flowing from your heart through your arms and hands and into the receiver. Trust the process of healing.

Allow yourself to so deeply merge with the healing energy flowing through you that you lose track of time and surrender to the process. (Pause two to three minutes.)

Visualize the receiver as completely healed, whole, and radiant with joy.

Before ending the healing, say a short prayer of gratitude, such as: I am grateful for the healing taking place now. I trust that it will continue in both visible and invisible ways, and that the will of God will be done in this situation.

Lift your hands slowly, shake them away from you, and then wash them in cold water.

Get both yourself and the receiver some room-temperature water to drink. Allow the person, child, or animal to rest as long as they wish before getting up.

When the adult or child arises, they may wish to share with you how they experienced the healing. Always allow them to share first. After they are finished, you may briefly share what you felt, as long as you keep it positive. After a healing, the receiver is still in a very open state and should only hear brief and positive feedback.

Laying-on-of-Hands
(Intermediate Form)

✤ *This meditation will guide you through the same laying-on-of-hands process as the basic form, with the inclusion of the receiver's head and feet and both sides of the body. Ask your partner what symptom or part of the body needs healing, so you know where to focus when you reach that location. The healing must be done with the person lying down, preferably on a massage table with a face rest. It also requires the healer to do a more thorough opening process of their own, spending a few minutes opening all seven chakras. Choose, with your partner, the color and healing symbol that you will image later in the meditation (see "Color Healing," chapter 1). This process will take about thirty minutes.*

If you are being healed, take your position on the table by lying face down. Take a long, deep breath and relax, consciously setting your intention to open and be receptive to the healing you are about to receive.

If you are the healer, place a pillow under your partner's ankles.

Make sure you know what symptom or part of the body needs healing.

Place a chair at the head of the table and sit down. The following instructions are for the healer.

Close your eyes, take a long, deep breath and relax. Allow your rational mind to take a rest during the count from ten to zero: ten–nine–eight–seven–six–five–four–three–two–one–zero.

Allow yourself to become aware of the light of Creation that is continually flowing down around and through you . . . . . . Breathe

. . . . . . See and feel this light and energy flowing in and out of all your chakras, front and back, as though your entire body is breathing this energy.

Feel it gently flowing down through your spine, all the way down your legs and into your feet . . . . . . Feel the energy in your feet connecting with the earth, down into the center of the earth's heat, and feel it flowing back up into your feet and legs, giving you a sense of grounding and stability.

Allow yourself to feel this light energy gently moving up your legs and into your first chakra at the base of your spine, gently opening the energy here in a spiral motion.

Feel it continuing to flow up in a spiral motion through your second chakra.

Into your third chakra.

Into your heart chakra, your center of love and compassion. Feel this light and energy gently opening your chest and heart in a circular motion . . . . . . Breathe.

Feel this sense of love and compassion filling your heart and chest and moving up into your shoulders and down your arms and into your hands . . . . . . As your hands fill with energy, feel it moving in a circular motion through your palms and down into your fingertips.

Now feel the light energy moving up into your throat chakra.

Into Your third eye.

And into your crown chakra, your center of spiritual consciousness.

Now that all your chakras are open and flowing easily with light energy, focus your attention once again on your heart chakra, and feel the light energy flowing gently in your center of love and compassion, and down through your arms and into your hands.

Now raise your arms to chest height and place your hands palm to palm about ten to twelve inches apart. Feel the energy between your two palms . . . . . . Breathe.

Slowly move your hands back and forth, and feel them filling with energy and warmth . . . . . . This is the energy of love, of creation, of healing. Feel it flowing through you.

In this healing process, we ask that our egos be put aside, our minds be at rest, and our hands be extensions of our heart, of our love, and of the Divine Light that flows through each of us.

We ask that this healing awaken us to the presence of God within, and the power of this Love to heal our hearts, our bodies, and our lives.

Now stand and move your chair aside.

Standing at your partner's head, very slowly and gently take your hands and place them as high over your partner's head as you can . . . . . . Drop all thinking and just feel, allowing your hands to slowly lower until you can feel the energy from your partner's head . . . . . . When you do, rest your hands in this position.

If the energy is comfortable, leave your hands here. Allow yourself to focus your attention on the flow of healing energy and love coming from your hands. If the energy is uncomfortable, raise your hands a little and gently pull upward with your hands, pulling out any energy that needs releasing from your partner's head.

Now raise your hands away from your partner's head, shake them out gently, and rub them together. Move to the location on your partner's body that needs healing. Place your hands as high over your partner's body as you can reach and close your eyes.

Slowly lower your hands until you can feel the energy from your partner's body . . . . . . Rest your hands in this position, feeling the healing energy flowing from your heart and hands.

Drop all thinking and allow your hands to intuitively respond. If your partner's body is releasing, allow your hands to pull energy upward. If not, feel the flow of healing energy from your hands moving down into your partner's body.

You may rest your hands in full contact with your partner's body if this feels appropriate, or if you wish, leave your hands above the body.

Breathe. Trust the healing process. (Pause one minute.)

Drop all thinking and just feel the flow of healing.

Now visualize the healing symbol and color your partner has chosen. Those of you receiving the healing can also visualize this symbol and color now.

The healer should softly say out loud: We accept the healing taking place now . . . . . . We accept the healing taking place now . . . . . . We accept the healing taking place now.

Focus all your attention on your hands. Breathe.

Those of you receiving the healing, allow yourself to trust the healing process and just receive this love and healing.

Deeper and deeper, feel the healing . . . . . . easy, gentle, flowing.

Now raise your hands from your partner's body, gently shake them, and rub them together.

Now, finally, move to your partner's feet.

Standing directly at the bottom of the table by your partner's feet, place both hands as high over their feet as you can . . . . . . Slowly lower your hands until they are poised above or resting lightly on your partner's feet.

Drop all thinking and feel the flow of healing energy balancing your partner's entire body.

Image the healing energies flowing all the way down through the body into the feet, and creating a strong stability and grounding in your partner's body.

Visualize the entire body as perfectly whole and healed.

The person receiving the healing can now slowly turn over onto their back. Remove the face rest, and place a cushion or pillow under their neck and knees if desired.

Ask if they are comfortable.

The healer should now move to the head of the table, stand comfortably with eyes closed, relax, and breathe.

Very slowly and gently, take your hands and place them as high over your partner's face as you can . . . . . . Drop all thinking and just feel, allowing your hands to slowly lower until you can feel the energy from your partner's face.

When you do, rest your hands in this position.

If the energy is comfortable, leave your hands here. Allow yourself to focus your attention on the flow of healing energy and love coming from your hands. If the energy is uncomfortable, raise your hands a little and gently pull upward with your hands, pulling out any energy that needs releasing from your partner's face.

Now raise your hands away from your partner's face, shake them out gently, and rub them together. Move to the location on your partner's body that needs healing. Place your hands as high over your partner's body as you can reach.

Close your eyes and slowly lower your hands until you can feel the energy from your partner's body . . . . . . Rest your hands in this position, feeling the healing energy flowing from your heart and hands.

Drop all thinking and allow your hands to intuitively respond . . . . . . If your partner's body is releasing, allow your hands to pull energy upward. If not, feel the flow of healing energy from your hands moving down into your partner's body.

You may rest your hands in full contact with your partner's body if this feels appropriate. If you wish, leave your hands above the body.

Breathe. Trust the healing process.

Drop all thinking, and just feel the flow of healing.

Now visualize the healing symbol and color that your partner has chosen. Those of you receiving the healing can also visualize this symbol and color now.

Focus all your attention on your hands. Breathe.

If you are receiving the healing, allow yourself to trust the healing process and just receive this love and healing.

Deeper and deeper, feel the healing . . . . . . easily, gently, flowing.

Now raise your hands from your partner's body, gently shake your hands, and rub them together.

Now, finally, move to your partner's feet. Standing directly at the bottom of the table, place both hands as high over your partner's feet as you can.

Slowly lower your hands until they are poised above or resting lightly on your partner's feet. Drop all thinking and feel the flow of healing energy balancing your partner's entire body . . . . . . As you stand at your partner's feet, visualize their whole body as perfectly whole and healed.

Focus all your attention on your hands. Breathe.

Those of you receiving the healing, allow yourself to trust the healing process and just receive this love and healing.

Deeper and deeper, feel the healing . . . . . . easy, gentle, flowing.

Knowing that this healing energy continues to flow in both visible and invisible ways, and trusting the healing process to continue, gently lift your hands from your partner's body. Step back from the table, take a deep breath, and gently shake your hands and rub them together.

The healer should softly say out loud: We are grateful for the healing taking place now.

As your partner continues to rest, wash your hands in cold water. Then get yourself and your partner each a glass of room-temperature water. When your partner feels ready, help them sit up and share with you how they feel. They should share first. Any sharing the healer does should be expressed positively and kept to a minimum. The person receiving the healing is in a very open and receptive state.

Encourage the person who has just received the healing to rest, eat well, and treat themselves with care for the rest of the day or evening. Suggest that he or she pay attention to any subtle sensations and changes in the body. Sometimes healing takes a few hours, or even days, to have its full effect.

Laying-on-of-Hands
(Advanced Form)

✤ *This meditation is similar to the intermediate form, but with the inclusion of all the patient's chakras and accompanying body locations. It is therefore essential that you have familiarized yourself with the chakras (see chapter 1), and used the basic and intermediate forms before you attempt this advanced form. Ask your partner what symptom or part of the body needs healing, so you know where to focus when you reach that location. The healing must be done with the person lying down, preferably on a massage table with a face rest. It also requires the healer to do a thorough opening process of their own, spending a few minutes opening all seven chakras. Choose, with your partner, the color and healing symbol that you will image later in the meditation (see "Color Healing," chapter 1). This process will require about forty-five minutes.*

If you are being healed, take your position on the table by lying face down. Take a long, deep breath and relax, consciously setting your intention to open and be receptive to the healing you are about to receive.

If you are the healer, place a pillow under your partner's ankles.

The healer should now place a chair at the head of the table and sit down. The following instructions are for the healer.

Close your eyes, take a long, deep breath and relax. Allow your rational mind to take a rest as you count from ten to zero: ten–nine–eight–seven–six–five–four–three–two–one–zero.

Begin with a prayer that is simple and appropriate for your spiritual beliefs, such as: I ask that my ego be put aside and that this healing be for the highest good of the person receiving it. I ask for God's healing love and power to be present.

Allow yourself to become aware of the light of Creation that is continually flowing down around and through you . . . . . . Breathe.

See and feel this light and energy flowing in and out of all your chakras, front and back, as though your entire body is breathing this energy.

Feel it gently flowing down through your spine, all the way down your legs and into your feet.

Feel the energy in your feet connecting with the earth, down into the center of the earth's heat, and feel it flow back up into your feet and legs, giving you a sense of grounding and stability.

Allow yourself to feel this light energy gently moving up your legs and into your first chakra at the base of your spine, gently opening the energy here in a spiral motion.

Feel it continuing to flow up in a spiral motion through your second chakra.

Into your third chakra.

And into your heart chakra, your center of love and compassion . . . . . . Feel this light and energy gently opening your chest and heart in a circular motion . . . . . . Breathe.

Feel this sense of love and compassion filling your heart and chest and moving up into your shoulders and down your arms and into your hands. . . . . . . As your hands fill with energy, feel it moving in a circular motion through your palms and down into your finger-tips.

Now feel the light energy moving up into your throat chakra.

Into your third eye.

And your crown chakra, your center of spiritual consciousness.

Now that all your chakras are open and flowing easily with light energy, focus your attention once again on your heart chakra, and feel the light energy flowing gently in your center of love and compassion, and down through your arms and into your hands.

Now raise your arms to chest height and place your hands palm to palm about ten to twelve inches apart. Feel the energy between your two palms . . . . . . Breathe.

Slowly move your hands back and forth, and feel them filling with energy and warmth . . . . . . This is the energy of love, of creation, of healing. Feel it flowing through you.

The healer should say silently: In this healing process, I ask that my ego be put aside, my mind be at rest, and my hands be extensions of my heart, my love, and the Divine Light that flows through me.

The healer should softly say out loud: We ask that this healing awaken us to the presence of God within, and the power of this Love to heal our hearts, our bodies, and our lives.

Now stand and move your chair aside.

Standing at your partner's head, very slowly and gently take your hands and place them as high over your partner's head as you can . . . . . . Drop all thinking and just feel, allowing your hands to slowly lower until you can feel the energy from your partner's head . . . . . . When you do, rest your hands in this position.

If the energy is comfortable, leave your hands here. Allow yourself to focus your attention on the flow of healing energy and love coming from your hands. If the energy is uncomfortable, raise your hands a little, and gently pull upward with your hands, pulling out any energy that needs releasing from your partner's head.

Now stand at your patient's left side. Place your left hand above the person's crown chakra and the other above the back of the neck. Your hands should be as far from the body as possible. Very slowly and gently lower your hands until you can feel the energy emanating from the body.

As it feels appropriate, you may lower your hands. Drop all thinking and just feel.

Now raise your hands, shake them gently away from you, and rub them together.

Place your left hand over the base of the neck where it meets the shoulders, and your right hand over the base of the spine, where the coccyx bone is located. Your hands should be as far from the body as possible. Very slowly and gently lower your hands until you can feel the energy emanating from the body.

As it feels appropriate, you may lower your hands. Drop all thinking and just feel.

Breathe . . . . . . Trust the healing process.

Drop all thinking and just feel the flow of healing.

Now raise your hands, gently shake them away from you, and rub them together.

Place your left hand over the upper back where the heart chakra is located, and your right hand over the sacrum, where the second chakra is located. Your hands should be as far from the body as possible. Very slowly and gently lower your hands until you can feel the energy emanating from the body.

As it feels appropriate, you may lower your hands. Drop all thinking and just feel.

Now raise your hands, gently shake them away from you, and rub them together.

Place both hands side by side over the middle of your patient's back, where the third chakra is located. Your hands should be as far from the body as possible. Very slowly and gently lower your hands until you can feel the energy emanating from the body.

As it feels appropriate, you may lower your hands. Drop all thinking and just feel.

Now raise your hands, shake them gently away from you, and rub them together.

Place your left hand over the back of the left knee, and the right hand under the left foot. Your hands should be as far away as possible. Very slowly and gently lower your hands until you can feel the energy emanating from the body.

As it feels appropriate, you may lower your hands. Drop all thinking and just feel.

Breathe . . . . . . Trust the healing process.

Drop all thinking, and just feel the flow of healing.

Now raise your hands, gently shake them away from you, and rub them together.

Move around to the other side of the table, and place your right hand over the back of the right knee, and the left hand under the right foot. Your hands should be as far from the body as possible. Very slowly and gently lower your hands until you can feel the energy emanating from the body.

As it feels appropriate, you may lower your hands. Drop all thinking and just feel.

Now raise your hands, gently shake them away from you, and rub them together.

At this point, keeping your voice low, suggest that your patient move down and turn over, so their head is resting on the table. Remove the face rest.

Place a pillow or cushion under the person's neck and knees, and ask if he or she is comfortable.

Now stand at the person's head, take a deep breath, and close your eyes. Once again, feel yourself getting grounded and comfortable. Bend your knees a little and relax your shoulders.

Place your hands side by side above the person's face. Your hands should be as far away as possible. Very slowly and gently lower your hands until you can feel the energy emanating from the face.

As it feels appropriate, you may lower your hands. Make sure to keep your hands at least one inch above the eyes. Drop all thinking and just feel.

Breathe . . . . . . Trust the healing process.

Drop all thinking, and just feel the flow of healing.

Now raise your hands, shake them gently away from you, and rub them together.

Move to your patient's right side. Place your left hand above the crown of the head, and your right hand over the third eye. Your hands should be as far from the body as possible. Very slowly and gently lower your hands until you can feel the energy emanating from the body.

As it feels appropriate, you may lower your hands. Drop all thinking and just feel.

Now raise your hands, shake them gently away from you, and rub them together.

Place your right hand over the throat, keeping your left hand above the crown. Your hands should be as far away as possible. Very slowly and gently lower your hands until you can feel the energy emanating from the body.

As it feels appropriate, you may lower your hands. Remember to keep your right hand at least one inch above the throat. Drop all thinking and just feel.

Now raise your hands, shake them gently away from you, and rub them together.

Place both hands over the middle of the chest, where the heart chakra is located. Your hands should be as far away as possible. Very slowly and gently lower your hands until you can feel the energy emanating from the body.

As it feels appropriate, you may lower your hands. Drop all thinking and just feel.

Breathe . . . . . . Trust the healing process.

Drop all thinking, and just feel the flow of healing.

Now raise your hands, shake them gently away from you, and rub them together.

Place both hands over the solar plexus, the location of the will chakra. Your hands should be as far from the body as possible. Very slowly and gently lower your hands until you can feel the energy emanating from the body.

As it feels appropriate, you may lower your hands. Drop all thinking and just feel.

Now raise your hands, shake them gently away from you, and rub them together.

Place your hands over the pelvis, the location of the second chakra. Your hands should be as far from the body as possible. Very slowly and gently lower your hands until you can feel the energy emanating from the body.

As it feels appropriate, you may lower your hands until they are about two inches above the pelvis. Rest them here.

Drop all thinking and just feel.

Now raise your hands, shake them gently away from you, and rub them together.

Place both hands over the first chakra, just below the pubic bone. Your hands should be as far from the body as possible. Very slowly and gently lower your hands until you can feel the energy emanating from the body.

As it feels appropriate, you may lower your hands until they are about two inches from the body.

Drop all thinking and just feel.

Breathe . . . . . . Trust the healing process.

Drop all thinking and just feel the flow of healing.

Now raise your hands, shake them gently away from you, and rub them together.

Place your left hand over the right knee, and your right hand under the right foot. Your hands should be as far from the body as possible. Very slowly and gently lower your hands until you can feel the energy emanating from the body.

As it feels appropriate, you may lower your hands. Drop all thinking and just feel.

Move around to the other side of the table and place your right hand over the left knee and your left hand under the left foot. Your hands should be as far from the body as possible. Very slowly and gently lower your hands until you can feel the energy emanating from the body.

As it feels appropriate, you may lower your hands. Drop all thinking and just feel.

Now raise your hands, shake them gently away from you, and rub them together.

Stand at the end of the table and place one hand over the top of each foot. Your hands should be as far away as possible. Very slowly and gently lower your hands until you can feel the energy emanating from the feet.

As it feels appropriate, you may lower your hands. Drop all thinking and just feel.

Now visualize the healing symbol and color your partner has chosen. [The healer softly says out loud: Visualize your healing symbol and color now.]

[The healer softly says out loud: We accept the healing taking place now . . . . . . We accept the healing taking place now . . . . . . We accept the healing taking place now.]

Focus all your attention on your hands. Breathe.

[The healer softly says out loud: Allow yourself to trust the healing process and just receive this love and healing.]

Deeper and deeper, feel the healing . . . . . . easy, gentle, flowing.

Image the healing energies flowing all the way down through the body, into the feet, and creating a strong stability and grounding in your partner's body.

Visualize the entire body as perfectly whole and healed.

Knowing that this healing energy continues to flow in both visible and invisible ways, and trusting the healing process to continue, gently lift your hands from your partner's feet.

Step back from the table, take a deep breath, and gently shake your hands and rub them together.

[Healer speaks out loud: We are grateful for the healing taking place now.]

As your partner continues to rest, wash your hands in cold water. Then get yourself and your partner each a glass of room-temperature water. When your partner feels ready, help them sit up and share with you how they feel. They should share first. Any sharing the healer does should be expressed positively and kept to a minimum. The person receiving the healing is in a very open and receptive state.

Encourage the person who has just received the healing to rest, eat well, and treat themselves with care for the rest of the day or evening. Suggest that he or she pay attention to any subtle sensations and changes in the body. Sometimes healing takes a few hours, or even days, to have its full effect.

Distant Healing

❖ *This meditation will assist you in sending healing to someone at a distance. The person may have a physical condition, or emotional, mental, or spiritual dis-ease. If it will help you to image, you may hold a photo of this person, or an object that belongs to him or her. It is best to do a distant healing at your meditation altar, or in a room where you can light a candle and be undisturbed. At the end of the meditation, wrap the object or photo carefully, and place it in a box or envelope.*

Find a comfortable position, either sitting or lying down. Uncross your arms and legs, and close your eyes. Take a long, deep breath, and let it out slowly. Allow your breathing to become full, deep, and relaxed.

As you count from ten to zero, allow your rational mind to rest, and you will become more receptive to the wisdom of your soul and its healing power: ten—nine—eight—seven—six—five—four—three—two—one—zero. You are now very deeply relaxed.

Focus your attention far above the top of your head, out into the heavens, and get in touch with a very brilliant, powerful, white light coming down to you in a stream of energy.

Allow this white light to flow all around you, and with each breath, allow it to flow into your lungs and through your entire body.

Now focus your attention on your heart, your center of love and compassion in the center of your chest. Image the white light gently flowing in a circular motion in your heart center, opening its energy.

As your heart fills with love and compassion, feel the strength of this energy in the middle of your chest.

Now image the person who needs healing as either sitting or standing in front of you. You may use a photograph, image the person in your mind, or repeat the person's name silently to yourself.

Breathe . . . . . . Feel this person's presence in front of you, and allow the white light to move out from your heart in a gentle stream of healing love across to the other person's heart.

Focus your attention on the person's heart, and image it filling with healing love and light.

Notice the change in this person's face and body as he or she begins to allow in the healing light and love.

The person's face may soften, the body may relax. Look into the eyes.

Image the light and love that is now in the heart begin to flow to all areas of the body.

Image this light and love spreading, cleansing, and healing this person's entire body.

If there is one location that especially needs healing, focus your attention there now. If the person's mind needs healing, focus the light in the head; if it is the emotions, continue to focus on the heart; if it is the body, focus on the physical condition.

See the healing energy and love as surrounding and permeating this area, gently bringing about healing changes.

If you are sending healing to a physical area, image healing taking place in the tissues, bone, and blood as needed.

Breathe . . . . . . Image this person as filled with light and love, new life, and strong energy.

Image the person as doing all the things he or she loves to do, and has always wanted to do.

On the count of three, image this person as completely well, healed and whole: one–two–three. Breathe.

See this person as filled with light and love inside, and surrounded with light and love for three feet all around.

Knowing that this healing and protection will continue, in both visible and invisible ways, give thanks to God for the opportunity to send healing.

Release any attachment or expectation you have about the results of this healing, asking only that God's will be done.

Gently release the person's image and the white light between your two hearts, knowing that you can renew this at any time.

On the count of ten you may open your eyes: one–two–three– four–five–six–seven–eight–nine–ten.

If you have been holding a photograph or object from this person, you may set it down and wash your hands in cold water.

Healing the World Soul

❧ *This final meditation gives you the opportunity to participate in the healing of the* anima mundi, *or world soul. In many ways human beings are like trees, with a central trunk, our torso; and branches, the arms and legs. We also have energy roots that extend down into the earth, and bark that protects us. The symbol of eternal healing is the Tree of Life, found within Genesis as well as the literature of other religions. This symbol shows us a way that we can actively join together for the healing of all Life. If you wish, you may sit outside with your bare feet in the earth.*

Find a comfortable position sitting with your feet flat on the floor or ground, and your arms and legs uncrossed. Close your eyes. Take a long, deep breath, and let it out slowly. Allow your breathing to become full, deep, and relaxed.

As you count from ten to zero, allow your rational mind to rest, and you will become more receptive to the wisdom of your soul and its healing power: ten–nine–eight–seven–six–five–four–three–two–one–zero. You are now very deeply relaxed.

Focus your attention deep within your heart, your center of love and compassion, and get in touch with the brilliant, powerful, white light within you.

Feel the gentle power of this light as it shines in the center of your chest.

This is the light of Creation, the seed of light planted within you by the Creator.

Image this white light gently flowing in a circular motion in your heart center, opening its energy.

Allow this white light to grow, and with each breath, allow it to flow into your lungs and through your entire body.

Image and feel this light flowing through your body like sap in a tree.

Feel it flowing up and down through the trunk of your body.

Feel it flowing out through the branches, your arms and legs.

Imagine yourself rooted in the earth, with this light energy pouring down into your roots. Feel your roots extending deep within the earth, and giving you a sense of grounding and safety.

Feel the white light energy flowing all around you, like nourishing and protective bark.

Feel it flowing out through your hands as your arms are outstretched.

Image and feel it freely reaching up toward the heavens through the top of your head, opening its light to combine with the light of all Creation. Breathe.

As this great light grows and expands, image your light reaching out to touch everyone and everything around you.

See it touching those you love, your home, your environment, your town or city.

Imagine yourself to be an enormous Tree of Life, spreading your branches of light and love, until they touch everyone and everything for hundreds of miles in all directions.

Feel yourself in the center of this circle of love, light, and healing.

Continue allowing the light to expand until it grows across continents and oceans, touching all the peoples of the planet.

Touch the rainforests, deserts, oceans, and lakes.

The animals, birds, plants, and trees.

Children being born and elders dying.

Feel the great size of your consciousness touching the planet with all the love that is in your heart.

And feel this love extending out to the moon, sun, and stars of our galaxy.

The moons, suns, and stars of all galaxies everywhere.

Feel the light of your heart as a healing beacon of love reaching through Eternity and touching all Creation. (Pause two to three minutes.)

Very slowly, as you feel ready, gently bring your consciousness and love-light back toward your center.

Very slowly return through the galaxies, this galaxy, to this planet.

Across continents and oceans, peoples and animal kingdoms.

Bring your consciousness and love-light back to yourself, your heart, your body. Breathe.

Allow yourself to sit as long as you wish in this deep state of love and light, and only when you are ready, you may open your eyes after the count of ten: one–two–three–four–five–six–seven–eight–nine–ten.

Namaste

I bow to the Divinity within you. *Namaste* is used for both a greeting and a farewell in India. The person speaking it brings their hands together, palm to palm in front of their heart, and bows to the other person. It is a lovely way to honor the Divinity within each other, and to remember our own.

Healing meditations are like seeds of light planted within your soul. If you nurture their potential, they can grow into a whole you. This takes time, commitment, patience, and self-love. Healing is a lifelong process. We all would prefer that it be instantaneous, but the beauty of the transformation is in the unfolding. Like everything in Nature, there is growth, change, abundance, and new life.

I encourage you to envision your life as a spiritual journey, and healing as a spiritual path. Once you choose the path, you have a direction for your journey. Everything that manifests along the path becomes an adventure and a new discovery. My students have sometimes questioned me about being a healer. Is it ever boring? Never. Each day brings new revelations and visions, deeper insights and healing, greater love and peace. The gifts of a rich soul are never boring. They are like buried treasure waiting to be unearthed and carried up into the light, where their brilliance can shine and remind you that you carry within the most powerful Healer of all. *Namaste*.

Acknowledgments

These meditations are really for my students and patients, who have listened with their hearts, and received them into their souls. To them I am deeply grateful. Many years of developing the TOUCHING SPIRIT® Training Program and countless private sessions helped facet these meditations. They have become like diamonds of strength and beauty, waiting to reflect each person's light back into consciousness.

My steadfast editor, Caroline Sutton, has contributed to this book's clarity, refinement, and design. I wish to thank Jackie Seow, the Art Director at Simon & Schuster, who has done a beautiful job designing the jackets of the hardcover editions of both *Touching Spirit* and *Seeds of Light*.

Nini Gridley, a faculty member of the TOUCHING SPIRIT® Training Program, read over the manuscript of *Seeds of Light* with great care and love. She made numerous and valuable suggestions as to content, style, and wording.

I am particularly grateful to Carolyn Reidy, the president of Simon & Schuster, who believed in both books and gave me the opportunity to manifest my dreams into reality. My agent, Lynn Nesbit, has supported this challenging process with grace and generosity of spirit.

As always, my mother, Karin Elizabeth Wallen Stratton, has provided a foundation of strength and love, without which I could not have become who I set out to be.

The Touching Spirit Center is located in Litchfield, Connecticut. For information about the Training Program, workshops, healing circles, and private sessions, you may call 860-567-0600, fax 860-567-5528, or write to:

Touching Spirit Center
16 South Street
P.O. Box 240
Litchfield, CT 06759-0240